Praise for

GETTING OFF

by Erica Garza

"The memoir shines light on the lonely (albeit impressively multi-orgasmic) world of a woman who binges not on food or pills, but on hookups and 'getting off.' . . . Her prose is appealingly no-frills and accessible. She writes like a . . . writer who knows better than to linger too long . . . over her memories—one who has learned the hard lesson that it is to keep the dangerous rushes of euphoric recall in check. . . . In reading Garza's insight into her own experience, we better understand ourselves. . . . The strong final chapters, sublimely set in Southeast Asia, are both inspirational and, dare I say it, still pretty kinky."

—*New York Times Book Review*

"Erica Garza has written a riveting, can't-look-away memoir of a life lived hard-core. . . . In an era when predatory male sexual behavior has finally become a topic of urgent national discourse . . . *Getting Off* makes for a wild, timely read."

—*Elle*

"Garza frankly and unflinchingly chronicles these experiences. . . . Garza's memoir is the rare sex addiction narrative from a female perspective, and a profoundly genuine, gripping story that any reader can appreciate."

—*Vice*

"Erica Garza's *Getting Off: One Woman's Journey Through Sex and Porn Addiction* is like *Belle de Jour* if Séverine was a real woman writing in the twenty-first-century and exploring her desires before she even had the chance to become a bored housewife. . . . That Garza's memoir ends with satisfying sex, sensuality, and self-acceptance is triumphant, but not because her prior sex life seems so licentious; there's plenty she *doesn't* do. Rather, the compelling part of Garza's story is that recovery entails the acceptance of her libido and refusal of shame. In a world that still fears female sexuality and buys into the dichotomy of the Madonna-whore complex, *Getting Off* is doing crucial work. . . . Garza is admirably bold, laying everything bare via her chosen genre. . . . If we care about the sexual health of our young people, we might encourage them to read *Getting Off*."

—*Los Angeles Review of Books*

"Accessible and intimate; her stories [are] relatable for anyone who has ever felt 'less than,' who has attempted (unsuccessfully) to fill the loneliness of life. . . . A heartbreaking and insightful read, a candid reminder that recovery is rarely a straightforward journey. . . . But it's hopeful, too—Garza is unflinchingly honest and introspective about her obsessions and how she found a path out of them. This is a necessary book that adds an important voice to a much-needed conversation."

—*Shondaland.com*

"For those of us whose understanding of sex addiction is relegated to a vague malady celebrities blame when they're caught with the nanny, Garza offers a sobering antidote. . . . This confessional memoir is peppered with statistics about porn use and sex addiction, and Garza's pull-no-punches style will twinge the sympathies of even the most prudish."

—*Booklist*

"[A] bracing chronicle of erotic dependency. . . . Exquisitely visceral and written with genuine emotion. . . . A provocative sojourn through the wilderness of sexual addiction."

—*Kirkus Reviews*

"[An] unflinching debut. . . . An honest voice to sufferers of sex addiction."

—*Publishers Weekly*

"Often, sex addiction is associated with the poor behavior of predatory men. Harvey Weinstein and Kevin Spacey claimed they were addicted to sex. In *Getting Off*, Erica Garza offers an important correction to that public narrative by telling her own story."

—Bitch Media

"Erica Garza's first memoir tracks her lifelong struggle with sex addiction, from 'strings of failed relationships and serial hookups with strangers, inevitable blackouts to blunt the shame,' shedding light on a very real dependency that women are rarely empowered to speak about."

—Glam.com

"What makes the book tick is Garza's ability and talent as a storyteller. She's a well-known essayist on this subject, and she is able to mine the depths of magic and mystery that makes sex what it is. . . . Painfully open and vulnerable. This memoir succeeds as the best memoirs do."

—*New York Journal of Books*

"Erica Garza's *Getting Off* is an unvarnished portrait of one the most difficult rooms to describe in the dark house of addiction; it is also a frank account of leaving. Garza does not make the escape look easy, nor does she give credit to one way out, but it is clear that the telling is an important part. For her. For all of us. As she describes so beautifully in these pages, it starts with pressing the bruise, locating the shame, and letting it go."

—Bill Clegg, bestselling author of *Portrait of an Addict as a Young Man: A Memoir* and *Did You Ever Have a Family: A Novel*

"In simple, elegant prose and with courageous honesty, Erica Garza traces the journey every girl must make toward womanhood: validating her own perceptions, admitting her own vulnerabilities and faults, trying and stumbling, learning to love and forgive herself and others. Yet somehow, Garza has turned this universal story into a page-turner. I read it in one sitting; I think you will too."

—Robin Rinaldi, author of *The Wild Oats Project*

"To speak about women's sexual desire as a singular thing, disconnected from male desire, is a transgressive and novel act. Add the ways Erica Garza admits to using her own pleasure to avoid genuine connection, and you practically have a revolution between these covers. With grace, humility, and lyricism, Erica Garza captures a rarely understood experience, and begins a different, badly needed discussion about women, sex, and addiction."

—Kerry Cohen, author of *Loose Girl: A Memoir of Promiscuity*

GETTING
OFF

ONE WOMAN'S JOURNEY THROUGH
SEX AND PORN ADDICTION

ERICA
GARZA

Simon & Schuster Paperbacks

New York   London   Toronto   Sydney   New Delhi

Simon & Schuster Paperbacks
An Imprint of Simon & Schuster, Inc.
1230 Avenue of the Americas
New York, NY 10020

First Simon & Schuster trade paperback edition February 2019

SIMON & SCHUSTER PAPERBACKS and colophon are registered trademarks
of Simon & Schuster, Inc.

For information about special discounts for bulk purchases, please contact Simon &
Schuster Special Sales at 1-866-506-1949 or business@simonandschuster.com.

The Simon & Schuster Speakers Bureau can bring authors to your live event. For
more information or to book an event, contact the Simon & Schuster Speakers Bureau
at 1-866-248-3049 or visit our website at www.simonspeakers.com.

Interior design by Carly Loman

Manufactured in the United States of America

3   5   7   9   10   8   6   4   2

The Library of Congress has cataloged the hardcover edition as follows:

Names: Garza, Erica, author.
Title: Getting off : one woman's journey through sex and porn addiction / Erica Garza.
Description: New York : Simon & Schuster, [2017] Identifiers: LCCN 2017013458 |
ISBN 9781501163371 (hardcover) | ISBN 9781501163395 (trade paper) Subjects:
LCSH: Garza, Erica. | Sex addicts—Biography. | Sex addiction. | Pornography.
Classification: LCC RC560.S43 G37 2017 | DDC 616.85/830092 [B]—dc23
LC record available at https://lccn.loc.gov/2017013458

ISBN 978-1-5011-6337-1
ISBN 978-1-5011-6339-5 (pbk)
ISBN 978-1-5011-6338-8 (ebook)

This book is for the wankers, the loners, the weirdos, the perverts, the outcasts, the bullied, the flawed, the awkward, the shunned, and the shamed.

"Ultimately, it is the desire, not the desired, that we love."

—Friedrich Nietzsche

PRELUDE

This guy I kind of know named Clay, who has a neck tattoo and sells arty photographs to tourists, is on top of me and he's not wearing a condom. I don't care. I'm completely sober. He's not.

I'm not sure what time it is. It is so dark outside that I can barely see Clay's neck tattoo, his condomless dick, or his mouth full of crooked teeth. I hear him grunting; I feel his body's weight—his six-foot-eight frame on my five-foot-two—and I know he's almost finished. I'm too tired to have an orgasm, so I wait for the inevitable end.

It's not that I don't enjoy this. *Enjoy* is not big enough a word. I have come to crave these nights with Clay.

Sometimes he calls during the day and we make plans to go out for drinks—never dinner, because what would we talk about? But then I don't hear from him until the middle of the night, when he's drunk or high and knocking at my front door. I don't care. I can't even picture him in a bar ordering drinks, sliding dollar bills over to the bartender, or making conversation with me fully clothed. It's true that I met him in a bar many months before, so I must have seen these things, but I was so drunk and heartbroken from my last breakup that I'm not sure exactly how that night went and what things he said to get me to swallow his cum.

He called me in the morning, and even though we made plans that I knew we wouldn't keep, I got dressed anyway and put on my mascara and took a small swig of the vodka I keep in the freezer to prepare myself for an awkward date, imagining the questions we'll trudge through out of politeness until the drinks we've ordered make us courageous enough to suggest the next move, to some-one's bed, likely mine.

After the time we'd chosen to meet had long passed, I wiped off my makeup, slipped on my pajamas, and fell asleep. Sometimes he shows up in the middle of the night; sometimes he doesn't. Either way I won't get another call for a few days, or a week, until he's bored and horny and we play this game again.

Tonight when I heard him knocking I woke up straightaway, but I stayed in bed a little longer than usual. For a fleeting moment I considered that letting him in might not be the best thing for me, which isn't so much of an *aha!* moment, but the usual com-mon sense that I choose to ignore. I thought about the sensation of his hips against mine; his heavy breath on my neck; the fullness that sex gives me, like having feasted on a hearty meal; but I also thought about the immediate emptiness that follows my nights with him or men like him.

I weighed the options like a sensible person. I did the expected. I took off my pajamas, opened the door naked, and led him back to my bedroom.

He turns me over, which is his favorite way to finish. My eyes, fully adjusted to the darkness now, focus on the dent forming between my headboard and the wall. I think about spackling. Then I see my reflection just above that, in the large mirror with a rattan frame that hangs above the bed.

I hold eye contact with myself while he fucks me, slipping into some sort of twisted meditation. I'm someone else, a queen or a goddess. He is just some lowly subject I use for fun. There are guards in armor waiting outside my door and maidens who will bathe me and rub me with sweet-smelling oils before putting me to bed.

But when Clay pulls out, he flips my body back over like a rag doll and comes all over my tits and stomach so a pool forms in my belly button and rolls out onto the bedspread.

Afterward, we lie there, our elbows touching. I am less sleepy than I was when I opened the door, so the awkwardness sets in fast. He asks how my day was, and then I wait in desperate anticipation for the *Call you tomorrow* or *See you in a few days*, which may or may not be true. I don't care. I dread the nights when he tries at intimacy, holds me in the sweaty crook of his arm for a few minutes before he retreats to the farthest corner of the bed to sleep while I lie there for hours, unable to sleep beside a stranger.

Finally he feeds me his lines and gets dressed and goes, and I give myself two orgasms in the wet spot of the bed. Once, to a three-minute clip of a teenage cheerleader fucking her stepdad on the kitchen counter while her mom showers upstairs, and then again to the thought of what a miserable slut I am to allow a guy like Clay to use me for sex.

There's nothing unique about this singular moment in bed with Clay. I can reach into my arsenal of memories and easily pick out another story just like it, sometimes not even including a man. Because what I got from Clay was more than just his penis inside of me. What I got was an elaborate mix of shame and sexual excitement I had come to depend on since I was twelve years old. And my methods of getting this only became darker and more intense so that it wreaked havoc on all aspects of my life until I became a shell of a person, isolated, on a path to certain destruction.

With Clay gone and my two orgasms over, I steep in the afterglow of having gotten what I needed. And, by now, I'm too exhausted to consider answering the overwhelming question echoing inside of me, where he and the cheerleader and the stepdad just were.

Why am I doing this?

What I block out of my mind, because it doesn't fit the sad story I'm devising in my head, is that I'm using Clay too. He's probably caught up in the same emptiness I am, desperately filling it with any warm body available. For what little conversation we have, Clay and I are actually quite similar, and we could probably have a genuine connection if we talked about these things. But we don't talk about these things because—well, it isn't sexy. I'd rather stick with the one thing that always manages to get me off—I'm bad, bad, bad.

introduction

THE SHAME ADDICT

My favorite porn scene of all time involves two sweaty women, fifty horny men, a warehouse, a harness, a hair dryer, and a taxicab. You can put it all together in a dozen different ways and I bet you still can't imagine just how revolting the scene actually is.

Revolting. I've been using this word and many adjectives like it to describe the things that have brought me to orgasm for more than two decades. I'm not just referring to porn scenes either. I'm also referring to those scenes from my own life, costarring semiconscious men in dark bedrooms and sex workers in cheaply rented rooms, where I prioritized the satisfaction of sexual release over everything else screaming inside of me *Please stop*.

Revolting: that summer after college when, after downing too many shots of tequila at a party, I stripped naked and took a bubble bath in front of a group of men.

Disgusting: slipping a few twenty-dollar bills to a woman who called me "baby" on the other side of a semen-stained pane of glass at a Times Square peep show.

Sickening: letting daylight dissipate and with it all my plans and obligations for the day because I'd rather stay in bed with high-definition clips of naughty secretaries, busty nurses, incestuous cheerleaders, drunk frat party girls, and sad Thai hookers.

I was thirty years old when I watched Steve McQueen's provocative film *Shame*, which stars Michael Fassbender as Brandon, a New Yorker whose sex addiction leads him to reject intimacy and seek fulfillment through sex with prostitutes and extensive porn watching.

There was something familiar in his story. But that wouldn't be a turning point for me. Not yet. It was more like an aura or a premonition, because over the next few years I would make many of the same mistakes I had made before, and I would make some new and more painful mistakes too, but right beside those mistakes there would be the hint of a growing awareness that can only come when you are in the midst of great change.

In 2008, three years before *Shame* was released, I was living in New York City with a man a decade older than me. We were engaged. He was a recovering alcoholic and went to meetings daily, sometimes twice a day, and I began to suspect that the primary reason for this frequency was to get away from me. And why wouldn't he want to get away? At that time in life I was racked with insecurity and relentlessly jealous. On top of that I was out of work and intimidated by his successful career as a filmmaker. He paid for everything, which seemed to make both of us increasingly uncomfortable over time. When I began to question his whereabouts and raid his journals for evidence of his presumed infidelities, he began to resent me. Eventually we fell apart. But one of the things I remember most vividly about our breakdown was his accusation that I was a sex addict.

"You're just saying that because you don't fuck me enough!" was all I could say, though I knew then, and I had known for a long time, that I *did* have a problem with sex. I just didn't know what to do about it. He suggested I go to Sex and Love Addicts Anonymous (SLAA) meetings, but I destroyed our relationship instead. It was easier.

I wouldn't go to SLAA for another five years, and when I did, I still wasn't sure that I belonged there. When people talked about the emptiness that came when they watched porn and how isolated they felt, I shifted in my seat and held my breath, feeling that same sense of recognition I had watching *Shame*. *Maybe these are my people*, I thought. But when an attractive and uneasy woman admitted to picking up a "few new STDs" at her latest orgy, I thought, *Well, I'm not that bad.* And I judged her and judged them and went home and masturbated.

◆

At thirty years old, at twenty-four, even at twelve, it was impossible for me to think about sexual pleasure without immediately feeling shame. I felt bad about the type of porn I watched. I felt bad sleeping with people I didn't like. I felt bad because of the thoughts I feasted on when I was having sex with people I genuinely loved.

For as far back as I can remember this is just the way it was. My sexual habits were sick and shameful. My thoughts were sick and shameful. *I* was sick and shameful.

But nothing would stop me from getting off. Even though I had a suspicion for a long time that this combination of pleasure and shame probably wasn't good for me, the satisfaction I felt in acting out was worth it.

That's why I was willing to do things like stick it out for six months with an alcoholic bartender even when he'd repeatedly piss the bed and forget to hide other women's clothes in his apartment. I didn't want to lose the easy, consistent access to sex and affection that being in a relationship guaranteed.

I would break plans with people who needed me—family members, friends—or not make plans at all, because I didn't want to miss out on any potential opportunity to have sex.

In Barcelona, suffering from what felt like the worst bout of strep throat I've ever had (which turned out to be mono), I chose to go home with the fifth guy in the space of a few weeks. It was the only thing I could do to stop thinking about the fact that I had just ruined a three-year relationship with the man I dated after the filmmaker, someone I truly loved and felt loved by, over a hand job with a Colombian man on vacation.

Instead of attempting to repair the damage, I slept with a French waiter who fucked me so hard I bled on his bed as if I were a virgin.

And then another French waiter, who took me to his friend's house instead of his own because his wife was there.

And then a Spanish guy, a German guy, and another Spanish guy. And I did it with the last one without a condom because who really cared at that point? Not him. Not me. I couldn't even moan or speak to him my throat was so flared up.

In those few weeks, it didn't matter who approached me. All that mattered was that I was approached. I didn't need an aphrodisiac-infused dinner, a long conversation spent bonding over our favorite writers of the twentieth century, or a glimmer of a potential future. All I needed was an invitation.

Don't get me wrong: judging someone based on the number of people they've slept with is absurd, and I know there are plenty of healthy, intelligent, and honorable men and women with strong sexual appetites. In some moments, with some partners, "sexually liberated" was exactly what I felt. But those moments were rare.

I'm much more familiar with the sad, anxious mess of a girl alone in her dark bedroom, hot laptop balanced on her chest, turning the volume down low, scrolling, scrolling, choosing, watching, escaping, coming.

I'm far too familiar with the girl who can't keep her hands from shaking or her throat from clenching, the girl who is just waiting for an invitation. Waiting for someone to show her some interest so she can put the loneliness away for a few hours and find some release.

Sometimes I wonder—if there had been more research and more discussion about sexual addiction in women,[1] would I have changed my behavior? Had there been more available examples of vulnerable, open, honest women sharing their journeys, would I have been more willing to embrace the possibility that I wasn't alone and unfixable? It's hard to know for sure.

What I do know is that isolation is damaging. Silence is damaging. And when you are isolated and silenced, all sorts of ideas, however twisted they may seem, can begin to seem real because they aren't ever dealt with properly.

I'll also admit that, while my misery was very real to me for a long time, I was willing to suffer the repercussions because the gratification of acting out was too good and I was hooked on a culture of chaos.

My adolescent years were convoluted with ideas that chaos was good, that depression meant you were a creative person. My heroes were Kurt Cobain, Courtney Love, Nancy Spungen. Sylvia

---

1 In 2012, *The Independent* (UK) ran a story called "Sexual Addiction: The Truth About a Modern Phenomenon," in which UK sexual psychotherapist Paula Hall noted an increase in clients seeking help for sex addiction. Hall found that out of 350 people who described themselves as addicted to sex, 25 percent were women and 74 percent of those women said they were heavy porn users.

fucking Plath. Little seemed cooler than Van Gogh cutting off his ear, than Virginia Woolf drowning herself. I romanticized brokenness as a means of resisting change, isolating myself, drinking too much, throwing tantrums, and playing Russian roulette with various dicks to make a point that I just didn't fucking care. I was a mess. I was interesting.

I filled journals with my depressed thoughts about my behavior, my loneliness, the hole I felt growing bigger inside myself, but I made no efforts to stop. If anything, all the brooding I did only intensified my habits, entrenched them. I would do everything I could to tear a relationship apart if the flip side meant having to deal with any real problem.

What began with harmless masturbation at twelve quickly became something more sinister. I wonder now if my parents suspected what I was up to all those hours behind closed doors with my computer. If they could tell by my exhaustion and dazed look that I had just binged for hours. But they never hinted at knowing. Do any parents confront their children about this?[2]

When I was living at home I'd take my laptop to my closet because I was afraid someone would bust through the lock on the door and catch me, or see me through the window that faced the street, even though I had blackout curtains and knew that was impossible.

Porn made me paranoid, but it was free and accessible and always effective. From watching soft-core on cable TV at twelve, to downloading photos at a snail's pace on AOL at fourteen, to tun-

---

2   The BBC reported in 2015 that of nearly seven hundred surveyed youngsters, ages twelve to thirteen, one in five said they had seen pornographic images that had shocked or upset them. They also found that 12 percent of those surveyed said they had taken part in, or had made, a sexually explicit video.

ing in to streaming sites with broadband forever after, my habit became more immediate, more intense, and harder to escape.

But what was I trying to escape? I had lived a pretty normal life, I thought. I had good parents who loved me the best they could, and I'd suffered no sexually traumatic events. Was I fundamentally flawed? This question led me, over the years, to a frantic investigation of my childhood journals, desperately trying to uncover some repressed sexual trauma that I could not find.[3] I threw my money at hypnotherapy, past-life regression, and other alternative treatments to find the missing link, eyeing my brother, my cousins, my uncles, my father, thinking, *Which one of you did it? Which one of you made me this way?* But when no such traumatic event could be found, the only thing left was that same unanswered emptiness and the conviction that I was inherently bad.

It wasn't until my early thirties when I finally started to realize that this problem wasn't just ruining my romantic relationships but *all* of my relationships—most notably, my relationship with myself. Because I had failed to examine all the reasons I had wanted to escape in the first place—the roots of my shame—I never developed the basic skill we all need to handle life's twists and turns: how to cope.

---

3   In the article "Sex 'Addiction' Isn't a Guy Thing" for *The Atlantic*, Tori Rodriguez points out that "exposure to pornography as a child was a stronger predictor of hypersexual behavior than sexual abuse as a child." In a 2003 study that compared rates of sex addiction among men and women on a college campus, researchers found that almost twice as many women as men fell into the "at-risk" categories.

one

THE GOOD GIRL

I grew up in the early eighties in Montebello, California, Southeast LA, where teenage pregnancy was on the rise and every Mexican restaurant claimed to have the best tacos north of the border. Living rooms were adorned with framed pictures of Jesus or the Virgin, and everyone believed in heaven and hell—not as abstract ideas, but as very real places. It was the kind of place where you could pick up your holy candles with your milk and bread at the local supermarket and you always knew someone celebrating a baptism or First Communion soon—giant events requiring ornate outfits and *tres leches* cake and a sense of relief on everyone's part that things were good with God, no one was going to hell just yet.

I rarely met anyone who wasn't Catholic. When it did happen, it was whispered about. *Did you know Mrs. Gonzalez is a Jehovah's Witness? Isn't that weird?* If you weren't Catholic, to whom would you turn for help? No priest? No Bible? It was unclear how a person could distinguish right from wrong without the Commandments. And I didn't even want to think of what happened to them after death. I imagined babies dying before they were baptized and shuddered at their unfortunate fates.

I often tell people now that I come from LA, or sometimes East LA if I want to hint at my Latino roots. LA is Hollywood glamour, money, and prestige; East LA screams danger, gangs, and irrefutable street cred. In truth, my life had neither. Montebello and all Southeast LA, home to cities like Bell Gardens, Pico Rivera, and Norwalk, were small, mediocre, boring.

My dad, a mortgage broker, helped low-income Mexicans buy first homes, while my mom, a housewife, made sure *our* home was intact. They balanced their checkbooks, and we bought clothes at Ross, and the only place we traveled to outside of the country was Tijuana, which my mom often said "didn't count" since it was only two hours south. My brother, Gabe, and I ran through sprinklers in the summer or laid down giant plastic trash bags for slipping and sliding. Katie Wilkins, a white girl, lived next door to us, which was rare in a predominately Mexican neighborhood, and I'd often peer at the swimming pool in her backyard from my bedroom window with envy. Mediocrity, which I felt was directly connected to my heritage, was my first source of shame.

But, in retrospect, we seem more privileged than I realized. I vacationed in Hawaii and Walt Disney World. I attended private Catholic school, from kindergarten through high school. My dad owned and ran a mortgage company for nearly twenty years until he sold it for a large sum and bought himself his dream car, a flashy Corvette that looked like the Batmobile, and a vacation condo in Maui. And by the time I entered high school we had moved into a house with a pool. I never knew what it was to go to bed hungry or face eviction, but shame has a way of being irrational. I looked at our life and I wanted more.

I simply couldn't understand why my parents would want to

live in such a boring place. There seemed to be nothing but strip malls and taco stands, nail salons and bail bonds. But to them, and to other Mexicans, Montebello was a big deal. In the late sixties and early seventies, when they were growing up, Montebello was nicknamed "the Mexican Beverly Hills." Housing prices were more expensive and the streets were safer than those in nearby East LA, where my mom spent her formative years. Tomas Benitez, the Chicano author and activist, said in an interview with LA's KCET, "Montebello was mythic when I was growing up in the 1970s. It was the place where middle-class Mexican-Americans lived and came from. It had that quality, if you could get out of East LA, Montebello was Nirvana, the promised land and Beverly Hills East all rolled into one location."

For my dad, who was born under modest circumstances in Mexico City and whose own father was an orphan, to be able to live in the Mexican Beverly Hills as an adult was a big step up. He played golf at the city's country club every weekend and served as an important figure in the city's Rotary International organization. We often ran into people who knew and respected him wherever we went—restaurants, the bank, the supermarket—and they'd shake his hand with sincerity, reassuring me and my older brother, "Your dad's a good man," in case we ever doubted it.

My mom, on the other hand, was less interested in the community. She often complained about the city's lack of good stores and its seemingly endless pavement. Sometimes she even complained about its propensity for attracting wetbacks, always laughing after this admittance, especially if my dad was around, before she'd lovingly touch his arm and coo, "Aww, I married a wetback."

That term *wetback*, coined from those Mexicans who illegally crossed the Rio Grande to get to America, was not an accurate description of my dad, who had crossed the border legally and traveled by road, not river. But that didn't stop my mom from muttering the word whenever she was feeling playful, or worse, when she was feeling wicked. Even though she has Mexican roots herself, I always thought that her teasing meant she considered natural-born citizens superior to those who had been naturalized. She would have likely picked this idea up from her own dad, a WWII veteran whose own parents were immigrants, and whose dark skin made him feel inferior in a country that was even harsher toward Mexicans than it is today.

The problem, for me, was that my neighborhood and my place inside it didn't resemble my preconceived notions of power. It didn't matter that my classmates at school shared the same Spanish-sounding last names and most of their grandmas didn't speak English either. I took note of the Mexican guy selling oranges on the corner, and the busboy picking up our dishes topped with messes of ketchup and crumbs, and I thought, *No, that's not me.* I even convinced myself now and again that I was superior to *those kinds* of Mexicans because my parents hadn't taught me Spanish. We were outgrowing our Mexican-ness, I thought to myself. Pretty soon it would be gone completely, forgotten like a dream.

My feelings of superiority never lasted long. I knew my classmates and I were part of a minority, and I didn't like the sound of that word, sitting heavy in my mouth and mind. I wanted to be like the blond-haired, blue-eyed Tanner girls on *Full House.* I wanted the calm, sensible family talks like the Seavers had on *Growing Pains.* I wanted a family tree that stretched back to Europe. Maybe England or Ireland, France even. But not Spain.

I got hooked on TV at a young age, marking the beginning of my intense bond with screens, and TV served as a window into the exciting world out there. I became obsessed with the families and neighborhoods I saw that were different from my own—which is to say, white. There was no George Lopez on TV then, no Sofia Vergara or America Ferrera. And I deemed the world "out there," on the TV screen and in the heart of glittering Hollywood, to be far superior to the Mexican Beverly Hills with its baldheaded gangsters, its teenage mothers, and its *paleta* men making their living selling sweet treats to kids on clean, suburban pavement.

Unlike my dad, who seemed perfectly content with his roots and his chosen city of Montebello, I leaned more toward my mom's chronic dissatisfaction and her fondness for escape. Like me, my mom also found herself captivated by screens. She loved foreign films—*Cinema Paradiso*, *Tie Me Up! Tie Me Down!*, *Shirley Valentine*—and I'd cuddle up with her on the couch for countless cinematic escapes, placing myself in the films and imagining the adventures waiting for me in adulthood.

Sometimes I would imagine taking trips with my mom. It's not that I didn't love my dad or that I wanted her to leave him forever, but maybe a few months? A year? I picked up on the tension that arose between my parents if my dad was working late again or on another client call. He usually returned from the office when we were already tucked into bed and was gone in the morning before we'd had a chance to get up, always trying to get ahead at the expense of my mom's growing resentment. My brother and I got used to having my dad around only on the weekends. But even then there were always more phone calls, more stacked files in front of him, and my mom found this difficult to accept, alternating between giving him the silent treatment and erupting in angry outbursts, depending on her mood.

My mom's moodiness became more pronounced as I grew older. Some days she'd park herself in front of the TV, bored eyes glazed over by some daytime talk show or murder mystery. Other days she'd take me to the mall to try on clothes and feast at the food court, deep-fried corn dogs with mustard and curly french fries. And yet other days she'd be annoyed by everything—the dirty dishes, the piles of laundry, her lazy children—and I'd think to myself, *She just needs a break. If we go away for a little while, she'll feel better.*

When my mom was upset, I sought solace in playing video games with Gabe, who was three years my senior. We spent hours toting machine guns in Contra, gobbling up mushrooms in Super Mario Bros., and scouring mythic lands for Zelda. I became obsessed with trying to beat him, frantically studying video-game magazines to learn the latest cheats, training myself not to blink, lest I miss a bullet or fireball and lose. When I wasn't playing, I was thinking of playing. When I was playing, I was thinking of what I'd play next.[4]

When we weren't saving princesses in front of the TV screen, Gabe and I were putting ourselves on the screen, acting out short films he wrote and directed—he'd decided early on he was going to be a famous filmmaker when he grew up. Gabe's gift for screenwriting and his skillfulness with my parents' camcorder earned him a lot of admiration. Family parties invariably involved the screening of a movie Gabe was making with my cousins and me as actors, typically toward the end of the night when our parents were tipsy and jovial.

I came to resent what I saw as Gabe's creative genius, even when my mom encouraged my rising interest in writing, buying me books and journals that I filled mostly with complaints about my brother intermingled with praise for all the boys I had crushes

---

4   Philip Zimbardo writes in *Man, Interrupted* that gaming and porn have the capability of becoming what he calls "arousal addictions," where the attraction is in the endless novelty and surprise factor of the content.

on at school. And whenever she caught me complaining about something being unfair, she'd murmur, smiling, "All the best writers had rough childhoods."

When Gabe didn't want to play with me, I'd terrorize him with kicks and shoves until he'd eventually shove me back, at which point I'd run crying to my mom in hopes he'd get punished. When she'd reprimand him, her long, curly hair shaking wildly around her face, I'd stand behind her, laughing and waving my hands at him, thinking, *I win! She loves me more than you!*

Despite my mom and dad's persistent praise of Gabe, I clung desperately to the idea that my mom loved me more. We were girls, after all, and this meant something. That's why she let me skip school and lie lazily in bed with her some days, watching movies and eating popcorn, saying, *Don't tell Dad I let you skip again.* I loved keeping secrets with her.

One night, when I was ten years old, my parents told us kids we'd have dinner in our fancy dining room. I was confused. My dad rarely made it to dinner. I thought the dining room was reserved for Thanksgiving and Christmas only. And were those candles?

I had heard the word *divorce* slither out of my mom's mouth on a few occasions when she was gossiping about my uncle's ex-wife, or when she was talking about certain kids' parents at school, and I wondered to myself if this is what was happening. Were my parents treating my brother and me to one final moment of togetherness before my dad packed up his suitcase? Would we be divided between them? Clearly I'd stay with my mom. And then, immediately after, *I wonder where we'll travel to first.*

"Your dad and I have some big news," my mom said, an excited smile on her face. A glass tumbler sat in her hand, filled to the brim with Pepsi and ice cubes, and she took gentle sips, letting suspense build around the table.

I looked at my dad, and he was smiling too.

"What is it?" Gabe said.

I kept my mouth shut, feeling excited yet guilty. Had I actually willed this into happening? Did all my imaginings of traveling the world with my mom come to fruition simply because I thought them? I considered the gravity of what this meant, that I had the power to destroy my parents' marriage with my mind. I pictured myself as some kind of witch, a source of power and wickedness.

"You want to tell them?" my mom asked my dad.

"OK," he said, and I held my breath.

"Your mom's going to have a baby!"

My mom exploded in giggles, the ice cubes in her Pepsi clanking against the glass while she stood up to give me and my brother kisses and hugs. But when she pulled me close to her, my face pressed against her cotton blouse, I burst into tears.

"Oh, baby, why are you crying? What's wrong?" She tried to pull away to look at my face, but I clung tight, digging my nails into her arm, refusing to let go. "Erica, what's wrong?"

I heard my brother laugh, confused by my reaction. And I felt my dad come over beside us and put his warm hand on my quivering head. But I didn't know how to explain the panic I felt at being cast aside, overshadowed by Gabe's talent and the importance of a brand-new baby, and so I lied when they asked again, "Erica, why are you crying?"

Finally, I answered, "Because I'm happy."

◆

I can remember, vividly, the sexual fantasies that bubbled in my brain, seemingly out of nowhere, during my mom's pregnancy. To distract myself from thinking about my new sibling, I turned my attention to other, more captivating places and daydreamed constantly. There's nothing like the bulging belly and emotional intensity of a pregnant woman to inspire curiosity about how it all works—babies, sex, the origin of life.

All I had ever heard about sex from my parents came from my mom when, passing the local high school, she pointed out a few pregnant girls who couldn't have been older than sixteen and said, "Don't ever let that happen to you"—and then, pointing to my crotch—"don't let *anyone ever* touch you down there."

My mom and dad both seemed uncomfortable when it came to addressing sex, and they were equally as aggressive about hiding it from me.[5] When things got hot and heavy in whatever movie we were watching, the response was immediate: "Close your eyes until we say," and I complied, listening to the indistinct sounds of what I was not allowed to see until it was all over.

I can understand my parents' reluctance at not wanting to talk about sex with me at ten years old, but "the talk" never came.[6] Sex

---

5   Advocates for Youth reported in "Parent-Child Communication: Promoting Sexually Healthy Youth" that many urban African-American and Latino mothers were reluctant to talk about sex with their preteen and early-adolescent daughters beyond biological issues and negative consequences. When maternal communications about sex were restrictive and moralistic in tone, daughters were less likely to confide in their mothers and sometimes became secretly involved in romantic relationships.

6   In a study by Kim S. Miller, Martin L. Levin, Daniel J. Whitaker, and Xiaohe Xu, called "Patterns of Condom Use Among Adolescents: The Impact of Mother-Adolescent Communication," when mothers discussed condom use before teens initiated sexual intercourse, youth were three times more likely to use condoms. Furthermore, condom use at first intercourse greatly predicted future condom use—teens who used condoms at first intercourse were twenty times more likely than other teens to use condoms regularly.

was something dirty and sinful, something to blush about, something to hide. These were obviously inherited ideas. My grandparents on both sides had the same reactions when a love scene unexpectedly danced across the TV screen: a shriek of discomfort followed by covered eyes and the demand that somebody *change the damn channel.* Whether it was a Latino thing[7] or a Catholic thing, I couldn't be sure. Even my teachers laughed uncomfortably and avoided eye contact when they explained that sex was something that happened "between two married people who loved each other," for one reason alone: procreation.

Though I had limited knowledge of how sex worked, I began gradually piecing it together when my parents weren't around. I'd been making lists of boys I wanted to kiss in my journal for a few years, but the lists became longer during my mom's pregnancy, and sometimes even included rudimentary drawings of body atop body next to the lists. There seemed to be no one I didn't find attractive in my fifth-grade class; I wanted all the boys—and some of the girls too—and even our teacher, Mr. Rivera.

In class, I'd stare at Mr. Rivera's crotch, trying to imagine what he looked like under his clothes. I stared at my female teachers' breasts and long legs. I stared at my classmates' bodies with such unquenchable curiosity and thirst, but I had no idea what to do with this desire except to try and ignore it, though the bubbling in my

---

7 The 2011 poll "Let's Talk: Are Parents Tackling Crucial Conversations About Sex?"conducted by Planned Parenthood Federation of America and the Center for Latino and Adolescent Family Health shows that out of 1,111 nationally representative parents of youth ages ten to eighteen, only 43 percent of parents were comfortable having discussions about these issues with their kids. The reason? Their own parents had failed to talk to them, thus perpetuating a cycle of misinformation or a complete lack of information altogether.

brain proved difficult to control. And since no other girls were talk-ing about this kind of thing, and I wanted desperately to be a good Catholic girl, I figured something terrible was happening to me.

Though I had attended Catholic school since kindergarten and weekly Mass was part of the curriculum, I didn't pray much. I made the sign of the cross with holy water, I closed my eyes and folded my hands so I looked like I was deep in prayer, and I con-fessed to the priest when required (always the same sins: *Bless me, Father, for I have sinned. I fought with my brother and I said bad words*), but these rarely felt like real acts of faith. They were obli-gations. My parents didn't pray much either. Not publicly, at least. For a short time, we attended Sunday Mass a few times a month, but then we turned into what my mom called "part-time Catho-lics," attending only during the holiest events, like Christmas and Easter. Pretty soon, we stopped going completely, so Mass felt like another school period. Despite this lack of practice, when I found out my mom and dad were having the baby, I started praying for one thing daily: *Please let the baby be a boy.*

I had to maintain my specialness somehow, and being the only girl seemed the best route. I was already used to being the only girl, not only of my immediate family but also among all my cous-ins. When Gabe wrote a new screenplay, I naturally got all the fe-male parts and I was the sole recipient of the kind of *oohs* and *aahs* that come with being the only kid wearing a pretty dress or sport-ing a new perm or having sparkly nails or whatever other girlie thing my mom bought for me that my aunts loved. I had a few fe-male younger cousins, but they were too little to prove what good and pretty and polite little girls they were. I had that covered.

I wrote down my favorite little-brother names in my journal—Freddy or Jason, because I loved horror movies—and I knelt at the foot of my bed in tireless devotion to God, whom I thought of as a magic genie then, thinking, *I will be a good girl forever if you grant me this one wish.*

But God showed me what he thought of my wishes when my mom brought home the shadowy sonogram print of her new baby girl.

"Look at your little sister, Erica," my mom said, handing over the picture. "Her name is Ashley."

I held the print in my hand, terror rising in my throat as I tried to make sense of the black-and-white blob, before somehow emitting a sound of false recognition. "I see her now. She's cute," I lied.

Mixed up in my feelings of jealousy, I also found myself contradictorily excited at the prospect of a protégé. If my brother didn't want to play with me, it wouldn't matter anymore because I would have my very own sister. I wrote letters to her, trying to psych myself up, but the clashing nature of my feelings only ever resulted in shame. I wanted desperately to silence my fears and be a good big sister, but I couldn't help this mounting anxiety from getting in my way.

I tried to keep things as they were before, asking to skip school so I could lie in bed with my mom and watch movies all day. She'd sometimes let me, but I felt our bubble already significantly altered and her attention hard to place. In bed with her it was hard to ignore the growing belly between us, the place where my sister now lived. And I couldn't help measuring myself against all the wonderful qualities I worried she'd have.

My body also experienced some scary changes around this time. I failed the vision test at school, and despite my desperate pleas that my eyes weren't *that bad*, my mom bought me glasses anyway. I also saw that I now had dark brown hair on my arms, where other girls in class had smooth, pretty arms. My mom then noticed that I was often coming home from school with scraped

knees and elbows from falling. When she took me to an orthope-
dic doctor and had me examined, his best diagnosis was clumsi-
ness. All these things seemed serious to me. I felt as if my body
were breaking down. I would be the ugly, nerdy, clumsy sister, and
thoughts of self-loathing filled my head.

When Ashley finally climbed out of my mother's womb that
September afternoon, my growing fears intensified. A baby needs
attention, after all, and as much as I tried to understand, my young
mind was shattered at how much attention she actually demanded.
My mom became fond of the camcorder, filming Ashley's every
move. My dad left work earlier to pitch in, and he spent lazy afternoons with her in the hammock that swung freely in the backyard
sunshine. When I'd shop with my mom and the baby, I might end
up with a blouse or pair of shoes, but if I noticed Ashley had more
items than I, I fumed. Everyone at the mall fussed over her chubby
cheeks and happy grin.

"Don't you just love your little sister?" they'd exclaim, and I'd
nod and produce an overly enthusiastic *Yes!*

Angry with my mom, my new sister, my brother, and my dad,
I decided to throw myself into my academics. I excelled in all my
subjects, especially language arts, and even found myself on the
spelling bee team, studying lists of words all day and often before
bed. I imagined myself becoming a national champ, my face on the
cover of *Time* magazine. I would become the family genius.

Placing myself under enormous pressure, I became restless
and squirmy. And I was nervous all the time. Nervous I would get
bad grades and be held back another year, which meant being held
back from the big, beautiful life I had planned for myself. Nervous
I would make my parents mad about something and be banished
to my bedroom without TV or books to suffer their worst punish-
ment: *Go to your room and think about what you did.* But I was

most nervous about upsetting God, the mighty ruler of the sky, more Nome King from *Return to Oz* than magic genie. If I upset God, then he would send me to hell, which was looking less like a fiery underworld and more like my bedroom in Montebello. For eternity.

My mom and dad were both impressed with my academic achievements, hanging up my Honor Roll and Student of the Month certificates on the fridge and proudly displaying my spelling bee trophies in the living room. I looked forward to after-school sessions with my fellow spelling bee enthusiasts, where we tested one another on words we didn't even know the meaning of, eating burgers and drinking chocolate malts while we nursed lofty dreams of academic stardom. I belonged to a clique of smart, sensible achievers, and I felt comfortable there. For a while.

It wasn't long before I noticed the intimacy of this clique and how the majority of the kids in class had no interest in words like *pirouette* or *precipice*. Their looks of boredom and back-row snickering were too intimidating to ignore, and so I purposely misspelled words and ignored my spelling bee comrades, becoming increasingly attached to a girl named Leslie, a popular tomboy who had blond hair and a surfer-dude inflection, despite her parents both being from Guadalajara, Mexico.

As Ashley grew into a little ball of energy and destruction around the house, tearing apart magazines and emptying drawers and cupboards out of curiosity while demanding every ounce of my mom's wearying attention, Gabe spent more time out of the house with his friends and returned only to retreat to his room or roll his eyes at any of us should we try to interact with him. I tried to stay out of everyone's way, continuing to excel at my academics in the most subtle way possible, so I didn't receive any loud praise from teachers. I threw myself into my friendship with Leslie full force. Everything my mom did annoyed me, and I mimicked the way Leslie talked to her mom, rolling my eyes and protesting at simple chores, to her dismay.

We spent weekends watching movies like *The Texas Chainsaw Massacre* and riding skateboards through the quiet residential streets of Whittier, where Leslie lived high up in the hills among big houses and hardly anyone spoke Spanish besides her family. I loved spending time in Whittier, and I wanted to hang out there all the time. Unlike Montebello, her neighborhood had antiques shops, a college, and white people. It wasn't long before I started listening to the same music as Leslie—Nirvana, Pearl Jam, and Smashing Pumpkins—dressing like her, and talking like her. When I spent the night at her house, we stayed up late watching MTV before falling asleep in her bed, our bodies close and warm like conjoined twins.

When I think about the term *first love*, it's difficult not to think of Leslie. My attachment to her was so intense, magnified by the urgency of youth, that the relationship still sticks out for me as one of the bigger ones in my life.

But I also recognize something dangerous and foreboding. I can't help but realize that this relationship became a model of unhealthy love. With Leslie, I learned what it was to rely too heavily on another person, besides my mother, for security and comfort. I felt, for the first time, what it was to be completely enamored of a person, how being enamored can trick the brain into thinking it's "in love," and how being in love can sometimes feel the same as being completely swallowed up by that love until all that's left when it's over is a gaping hole just waiting to be filled again.

two

THE WEIRD GIRL

My newfound interest in rock music led me to LA's alternative radio station KROQ, which I listened to all day. If I stayed up late enough, I could also listen to the radio show *Loveline* at night. Hosted by Dr. Drew Pinsky and Adam Carolla, the syndicated program offered medical and relationship advice to listeners, and often had actors and musicians as guests.

Dr. Drew would, in later years, be applauded for his work on sex addiction, but it was *Loveline* that first introduced me to masturbation, which would soon become my primary method of acting out.

I was twelve years old when a caller fascinated with water faucets—a woman—called in and gave me an outlet for all my pent-up sexual frustration. She'd discovered this new and gratifying way in which to have mind-blowing orgasms. I had no idea what an orgasm was, but hearing the way she talked about it, I now *needed* to know. She said all she had to do was sit in the bathtub, spread her legs, and turn on the water faucet.

I could do that.

There are some things in life you don't remember, no matter how hard you try. Either they have no significance to us or they have too much that we couldn't bear to carry the burden of so much meaning every day. And so we make stories and construct memories of half-truths to try and make sense of it all. I wish I remembered the moment I tasted chocolate for the first time. Did it have the bitterness of high cacao? Or was it milky and sickly sweet on my tongue? What was it like when I first saw the sea? Did my stomach tie itself into a knot in the presence of such vastness? Was I overcome with delight? Did I laugh? I have no idea.

And then there are those things we cannot forget, memories we play over and over in our heads because they have a history of significance in them—they make us who we are. I remember my first orgasm in more profound detail than what I did just moments ago. I remember the chill on my dry kneecaps, pressed up against the cold walls of the bathtub while the steady stream of warm water plummeted to that untouched space between my legs. I remember the dried spots of mildew in the corners of the tub and how my own reflection bounced back at me from the metal faucet, warped and unfamiliar. I remember the light flickering above me, the consistent buzz of the bathroom fan and the muffled sounds of the TV from downstairs. And, catastrophically, I remember the pleasure. A singular kind of pleasure that has haunted me ever since, forever inimitable no matter how hard I try to find it again. Followed by immense fear. *What was that? Was it normal? Is something wrong with me? Should I do it again?* Yes. Absolutely. Of course I did it again. And again. The bathwater went lukewarm, then cool. I remember the goose bumps popping up across my body like I were covered in a sheet of bubble wrap.

I became extremely fond of long baths. My mom often interrupted my sessions of bliss by banging on the door and shouting out, "Are you still alive in there?" Exasperated—my developing chest blotched red with satisfaction, my pruney fingers clinging to the edges of the tub—I'd call out, cheerfully, "Yup," and go at it again. I was most definitely *alive*.

Although I felt alive and excited and, most significantly, *relieved* at having found my outlet, I also felt guilty. My first orgasm brought with it an equal balance of pleasure and mortification. Only that pleasure lasted mere seconds until the next time I masturbated, while the mortification lasted. And lasted.

I hadn't even gotten my period yet.

◆

Every year, since kindergarten, we had our backs examined at school. You stood in line, waited for your turn, bent over, and went back to class. It was a nice break from schoolwork, but I wasn't sure why they made such a big deal about it. No one ever got pulled aside and told something was wrong. Except that one year. Seventh grade. When they pulled me aside.

Terms like *scoliosis* and *major curvature of the spine* fell from the lips of a kind-eyed, smiling Indian man Dr. Dayal. Prompted by the examination at school, my parents brought me to his office for a proper diagnosis. Human skeletal replicas in various degrees of severity stared back at me, slumped over in my seat, and terrified. When he said the word *bracing*, I sat straight up.

After a few more visits, Dr. Dayal condemned me to wear a Boston brace, a clunky metal and plastic contraption that weighed down my body from the neck to the hips, for two whole years, only removing it for bathing.

"You can wear it under your clothes," he assured me when my eyes welled up in tears in his office. I looked down at a scoliosis pamphlet, where a braced girl around my age smiled up at me. She wore her brace on the outside of her clothes, which I thought was complete lunacy.

My mom and dad were already asking about alternatives, but there seemed to be only one.

"We can perform corrective surgery," Dr. Dayal offered. "In fact, we may have to anyway, if the bracing proves unsuccessful."

Being fitted for the brace involved many more visits to Dr. Dayal's office for examination, but the part I dreaded most were the X-rays. I stood barefoot in the paper-thin X-ray gown, waiting anxiously as the technician and the doctor examined the illuminated black-and-white sheets of my spinal column in the other room. I remember the tingling sensation at the back of my throat, the hollowness of my belly, the visceral sense of impending doom. I was certain that, at any moment, Dr. Dayal would emerge to tell me that my spine had grown crookedly because I had masturbated too much.

How else to explain the awkward question mark growing inside my body? I could think of nothing to blame but my frequent baths. Maybe the hot water and the way my body contorted at orgasm had resulted in this. What would my parents say?

Wearing the brace wasn't exactly painful, at least not physically. But it was definitely awkward. Something so simple, like dropping my pen in class, now required more effort than ever before. I couldn't just bend down to quickly retrieve it. I had to get out of my seat and get down on the floor as if I were crawling for it. Then I'd have to hang on to the desk or chair to pull myself back up, but sometimes I'd lose balance and slip. At home, getting up in the morning was also a step-by-step process. I slept on my back—the only comfortable position with a clunky brace— and to get up, I had to roll over to one side, push my body up with all of my arm strength, and swing my legs around. Always in this order, and carefully. Having so much plastic and metal against my body also left me sweaty, uncomfortable, and hot all the time.

Where I may have already been shy at school, I now became extremely withdrawn. I was terrified classmates would make fun of me, so I avoided social interaction as best I could. I was sure most students knew about my brace, since the teachers knew and I often skipped PE class, but no one had actually confronted me about it and I needed it to stay that way. I hardly spoke in class and skipped school often, blaming my back problems.

The more introverted I became, the cooler Leslie appeared and the only normalcy I saw in my life was in maintaining our friendship.

One Friday, Leslie showed up to school without her usual ponytail. She'd cut her hair into a bob, longer in the front and parted down the middle. I watched, enviously, as our classmates complimented her, and I made a mental note to get the same haircut on the weekend.

That weekend was pure joy. With my new bob, I looked exactly like Leslie and felt like a new person. A *better* person. I imagined myself confidently strutting the school corridors. Boys would whistle, teachers would nod in recognition, and all the popular girls would want to be my friend. Leslie and I would be the coolest girls in school—a power duo—and cute white boys would pick us up after class and take us to band practice with them.

When Monday came, I had butterflies in my stomach on the drive to school. My mom was happy. It was the first time I was in a good mood since being braced, and she further stoked my ego by complimenting my hair.

When I entered the classroom, smiling, I ran straight over to Leslie's desk to show her my new cut.

"Check it out!" I said. "I cut my hair!"

Her eyes widened when she saw me. "Are you fucking kidding me?"

"Huh?" I said. Her reaction confused me.

The boys she'd been talking to exploded in laughter, and one of them yelled, "Oh shit, Leslie! You have a biter!"

"A what?" I looked at him uncertainly.

"A biter," Leslie snapped as she stood up from her seat. "You totally copied my hair and it's not fucking cool." I saw tears come to her eyes, which took me by surprise. "Get out of my face," she said.

I wanted to cry too. Shocked and paranoid, I slunk away from her, made my way to my seat, and opened up my book to pretend I was reading. My heart thumped against my chest. I hadn't even considered the possibility that Leslie would be mad about the haircut, and I definitely hadn't considered ever losing her as a friend. Who would I hang out with now?

Those next few weeks, I hung out with nobody. When I came into class, I found notes on my desk with the word *biter* scrawled across in big letters. Leslie and her friends randomly yelled the word when it was quiet in class, and everyone would laugh. Once, after using the bathroom, I came back to find that all my textbooks and notebooks had been removed from my desk and backpack and scattered across the floor. Someone had even stolen my lunch. As I picked up my things and put them away, I heard Leslie and her friends snickering and giving high fives from the back of the room. The teacher apparently hadn't noticed any of this.

I would often spend lunch at the nurse's office, complaining of headaches. The nurse, a young woman with freckles across her nose and a soft voice, became my savior. She let me eat my lunch there among clear jars of cotton balls and endless boxes of Band-

Aids just so I wouldn't have to go outside. She never asked me why I preferred to eat there, and for this I was grateful. I didn't want her or anyone to know what was going on.

But everyone knew that since Leslie wasn't my friend anymore, I didn't have any friends. So along with the word *biter*, they started calling me "loner." Around this time, I skipped more school, not giving my parents the details, though I'm sure they figured out what was happening when phone calls and invitations for sleepovers stopped coming. Teachers also must have known what was going on, but nobody at school tried to intervene. When my parents asked me if I wanted to switch schools, I politely declined. If I agreed to this I thought I would appear weak in the eyes of not just my parents but Leslie and her friends too. And though I felt weak and broken inside, I kept those feelings a secret.

I couldn't have known then, and it would take years before I'd figure it out, but the emotional distress I was experiencing as a result of scoliosis was actually not that unique. Had I been part of a support group, or had there been a hotline or some TV show with a back-braced kid as its protagonist, maybe I would've found some comfort. But all I felt was odd and alone.

It's not that my family didn't want to support me—I just don't think they knew how. The only time my mom explicitly addressed the situation, I was sitting in my room alone doing my homework. All she said was, "In a few years, none of this will matter. They'll still be the same miserable people, and you'll be doing amazing things. I promise you there's a bright side." And knowing how keen I was on keeping a journal, she encouraged me to write it out. Always: "Write it out, Erica. That way it's out of your head and onto the paper." I wanted to believe in the bright side she spoke of, but I was doubtful.

My mom and dad weren't big on therapy. They'd only once

sought outside help during a rough patch in their marriage, but it was with a priest a half-hour drive away, where they wouldn't risk running into somebody they knew. And it was short-lived. Marriage counseling, or any other type of therapy, was for genuinely damaged people, not them. Something only rich white people did in movies, sprawled out on a recliner, complaining about meaningless, self-indulgent things. My dad was more inclined to read Dale Carnegie. My mom was more inclined to pretend everything was fine, or that it would be soon enough. I've often wondered what would have been prevented in my life, what habits I wouldn't have picked out, and what men I wouldn't have picked up had I simply gone to see a therapist early on and learned to manage the emotions that were rising up in me in alarming disarray.

Instead, all I could do was blame everyone, especially God.

Throughout the rest of my years in junior high, I spent my days alone, writing in my journal and listening to angsty music. And more fervently than before, I masturbated. Not just reserved for the bathtub anymore, I masturbated when I got home from school, before dinner, after dinner, and soon found that I couldn't even fall asleep without an orgasm. Dredging through the book *Treasure Island*, I remember making a deal with myself to masturbate to orgasm at the end of each chapter so I could finish reading by the due date. There are thirty-four chapters in that book and, once I made that deal, I enthusiastically, yet guiltily, breezed through them over the course of a few days. Robert Louis Stevenson will always be an erotic novelist in my mind.

My hormones were a freight train. I tried to keep up. I wonder now if I would have eventually lost the thrill of masturbation, but I found new thrills. I started staying up late, when my mom and dad were snoring away in oblivion, to watch soft-core porn on Cinemax. Shannon Tweed became my nighttime hero. I didn't know whether to hate her or love her, but I knew I needed her. During the day, I made other arrangements. I'd wait for Gabe to leave the house and then I'd raid his stash, hidden in his bedside drawer under men's fitness magazines and school notebooks. Dirty magazines. Unlabeled VHS tapes. I masturbated every day, multiple times a day, until I was exhausted and sore.

I couldn't have dreamed up a better solution to the endless ache of my rushing hormones than the endless novelty that would become my burden, and equally my passion, encapsulated in the static buzz and endless stretch of dial-up internet.

three

THE SICK GIRL

Some days I was 16/F/LA with blond hair, blue eyes, long legs, and C cups. My name was Emily. Other times I was Jacqueline, 22/F/NY with red hair, green eyes, a tiny waist, and D cups. I liked wearing lace teddies, fishnet stockings, and stilettos. I loved nine-inch penises, being fucked really hard, being eaten out, my clit nibbled. Sometimes I preferred fucking on countertops, other times office desks.

My online sexual proclivities began with chat-room encounters when I was thirteen. Dial-up internet in 1995 didn't offer the same instant access to streaming porn clips so common today. Clips took hours to download, sometimes even a whole night, and they weren't easy to find.

Before AOL became my go-to for browsing, there was the Imagi-Nation Network, a.k.a. the Sierra Network. It was an online multi-player gaming system that allowed users to create their own avatars and play trivia or cards with other users. You also had the opportunity to "cyber" with strangers, which meant have virtual sex through text. Suddenly, erotic reading took on a whole new demeanor.

I sat on the edge of my dad's ergonomic swivel seat, desperate for the conversation prompt A/S/L (age/sex/location), which was typically followed with "What are you wearing?" *A lace thong.* "What's your bra size?" *36D.* "What do you want me to do to you?" *Anything you want.* And on and on. Of course I wasn't wearing a lace thong, and my tits were not even close to 36D, but none of that mattered. Soon I was the one A/S/L-ing my way around the digitally provocative online community, tricking my parents into thinking I was only playing checkers with other kids around the country.

A lot of these encounters were random. I cybered with users who said they were twenty-year-old males as enthusiastically as those who said they were forty-five. I cybered with so-called females too. I always lied about my age, usually saying I was sixteen, which neither the twenty- nor forty-five-year-olds minded. Maybe they were lying too.

The more versed I became in cybersex, the more I learned about how the act worked, but it would still be years before I would experience anything remotely close to it in real life. I figured that when the time came, I'd be sufficiently prepared.

In addition to random encounters, I also had regulars. There was Jeff, a thirty-two-year-old from Miami who liked fucking on his desk at work—he'd mention the stapler, the keyboard, and other office supplies to set the scene. There was Kyle, a twenty-five-year-old from Chicago who described us fucking on elevators, in closets, and in other tight spaces.

I started off submissively, answering a mere *yes* or *no* to any of their requests, and offered only slight descriptors about my imaginary appearance. But as time went on, I picked up words like *cock* and *blow job* and *cum* and started to piece these things together.

Back in the nineties, we had one shared computer in the living room, and so these sexual adventures took place out in the open. This meant having to become very familiar with screen minimizers and the escape key. Soon I was excellent at typing rapidly and efficiently. Even now there's something erotic in picturing the dark blue sofa that sat adjacent to that old computer desk, those white shutters just behind the monitor, and the whirring of the air conditioner from the other side of the wall. Every creak I heard in the hallway that could've been my mom or dad walking in to catch me would send me into an adrenaline frenzy.

Using this computer meant that I couldn't always masturbate right away, at least not during the day, because there was always somebody hanging about. I had to wait to masturbate later in my room or in the bathroom. This delayed gratification always led to bigger, more mind-blowing orgasms later when I was able to relieve myself, and so I was more or less fine with my situation. But I preferred having cybersex late at night when everyone was asleep. If I had enough time, I could even sneak over to the TV and squeeze in some late-night programming, that coveted SSC warning label flashing before the movies began, signaling strong sexual content.

When the ImagiNation Network went out of business, my parents signed up for AOL, and with speeds improved and what seemed like endless chat rooms, I rarely felt lonely when I was logged in. Chatting and having cybersex assured me that, even though I had few friends in my real life, I had friends *out there*, and how similar we were!

When I wasn't staring at screens, I was staring at pages. Heavy reading encouraged heavy writing, and I read everything, from our encyclopedias—I'd randomly pick a letter and a page and submerge myself—to my mom's collection of biographies. I especially liked reading about exotic, faraway places: Venice, Tokyo,

Texas. Everything outside my city seemed exciting in my young and naive mind.

If there was a strong female protagonist in a story, I liked it. If there was a female protagonist with complex problems, I liked it more. I remember picking up Deborah Spungen's memoir *And I Don't Want to Live This Life* about her daughter, Nancy. The book followed Nancy's tumultuous childhood and adolescence into her young adult years, when she fell in love with Sid Vicious of the Sex Pistols, got hooked on heroin, and eventually died at his hands. It was probably the first time the notion of violent romance seemed enticing to me. Another favorite was a circus-oddity picture book called *Very Special People*. This book I kept by my bed. I flipped through the images of dwarfs, giants, the conjoined, and the hairy, feeling an odd sense of comfort and twisted connection.

◆

In the eighth grade, my dad's youngest brother, my uncle Mario, moved into our house with my two cousins Mario Jr. and Jake. Uncle Mario's wife had left him years before, and my uncle often had trouble making ends meet and keeping a stable job. This resulted in many eye rolls and disapproving sighs from my mom, who blamed my uncle's lack of discipline for his financial instability and resented my dad's consistent willingness to help his little brother out.

Already accustomed to my brother ignoring me, I now felt even more excluded when I saw the boys in their tight little pack, shooting hoops in the backyard and going "for walks," which meant heading to the local park to smoke weed under the trees. I'd press my ear against my brother's bedroom door when they were in there together, my heart thumping, my palms clammy, hoping they'd hear me and ask me to join them so we could all share inside jokes like we did before I was braced and I became this weird, lonely, masturbating creature. But I never knocked, and I'd only occasionally hang out with Jake, who was a year younger than me.

Sometimes Jake and I would pretend we were in a band together and set the camcorder up on its tripod to film music videos in our garage against a cluttered backdrop of my dad's old work files and laundry baskets filled with unused hangers. I blasted Nirvana or Hole CDs on the stereo and strummed along with the bass my parents bought me for my thirteenth birthday, while Jake banged on an upside-down bucket with rulers. But he often looked bored, and I began to think he only spent time with me because he pitied me. This made me feel terribly insecure and eager to impress him, buying him CDs and candy with my allowance money and feeding him compliments to get him to stick around. But the pack of boys usually won out, and, despite my efforts, I often felt him pulling away.

"Do you want to play music in the garage?" I'd ask him casually, so he wouldn't sense my desperation and think I was too clingy.

"Not today" became his usual response, and then just "Nah," while he looked away from me and over to the TV or anything more interesting. If he seemed bored and disengaged, this changed in an instant when the guys came into the room or called him over to join them. I couldn't blame him. I wanted them to call me too. I wanted to smoke pot and skip school and tell jokes. I always laughed loudly when one of them told a funny story, and I never protested when they changed the channel to something they all wanted to watch, even if I was already enthralled in a movie. But I still wasn't part of their pack, and it became obvious to me why: my vagina.

With my uncle and cousins in the house, my mom now had five

kids to take care of, including a needy toddler, and seven people to feed (eight including herself), and she found herself more overwhelmed than ever. Every few weeks her fury would lead her to pack up her suitcase and roll it over to my bedroom door.

"We're leaving in twenty minutes. Pack your bag and don't forget your toothbrush." Ashley would be on her hip and she'd have a look of determination on her face, one that said, *I've had enough.*

We never went far. At the local Sheraton, we'd get a room with one giant bed and more pillows than we knew what to do with, and best of all, pay-per-view movies. I'd dive into the bed as soon as my mom swung open the door to our perfect pocket of life for the next few days.

"Get whatever you want from room service," she'd say, and I'd order a feast. A shrimp cocktail with extra cocktail sauce, breaded chicken strips with fries, and a hot-fudge sundae. If I couldn't wait until the food arrived, I'd pop open the minifridge and devour the Snickers bar and a can of Pepsi.

The hotel room always had a big bathtub in the bathroom too, so I'd soak in bubbles and masturbate quietly as my mom watched TV, careful not to move my hand too rapidly and splash the water around.

Elsewhere was *happy*. Mom felt it too. She seemed relaxed and even cheerful in that hotel room, clicking through pay-per-view movies, flipping through the room service menu, and rummaging around the minifridge.

When our getaway was over, I shared my mom's dismay in having to return home. Seeing her resigned to the kitchen and piles of laundry, I wanted desperately to make her happy but didn't know how. I now fantasized about her leaving us all behind, not just for quick getaways to the Sheraton but to some other life, like the woman in *Shirley Valentine*. Now I understood why it was her favorite movie. Shirley Valentine ran away. Being a housewife sucks.

I often thought about approaching my mom with the idea, to let her know we would all be fine if she needed to leave and that I wanted her to be happy. But navigating around her moods and trying to avoid an unfavorable reaction took precedence. I didn't want her to think I *wanted* her to leave. I kept my fantasies to myself.

◆

When I was fourteen, Dr. Dayal finally freed me of my brace and surgically straightened out my spine during my freshman year of high school. Part of the procedure included removing nearly all my spinal discs and a left rib. The rib was then fused to my spine along with two titanium rods, permanently preventing me from back bending and requiring intense physical therapy for months. I have two huge scars: the vertical one that runs from the base of my neck to my sacrum and the horizontal one right below my left rib cage.

I didn't mind skipping some months of school and going into surgery, and I definitely wasn't scared of the pain when Dr. Dayal told me I would be hooked up to a morphine drip for days and then switched to Vicodin for months. The idea of drug use, even for medical necessity, was the definition of cool at that fragile age. I hadn't yet experimented with any drugs, but most of my cousins, my brother, and many of the writers and musicians I admired had experimented or even become addicted. Drugs and creativity were then unavoidably linked.

Getting a new back seemed appropriately timed, as it aligned with my new desire to reinvent my identity. Losing the brace helped free up my wardrobe constrictions and I experimented with my look, from punk to goth to rockabilly. These were crucial changes from my uniform of oversize rock band T-shirts and bulky sweaters. My focus then turned to beautifying my body. Grooming took up hours of my time, whether I was getting ready to go somewhere or not. I also developed a preoccupation with body hair, shaving and plucking and picking at any patch of hair I saw on my body that wasn't on the top of my head.

My private high school was a fetishist's dream. With its plaid skirts, knee-high socks, nuns in habits, and a pervading atmosphere of innocence and sexual repression, high school took me away from everyday interaction with boys around the same time I started to have a genuine interest in them. I had been hungry for sexual intimacy for years, but from a safe distance. The thought of having sex, fondling, or even just kissing intimidated the hell out of me. But my curiosity was winning out. I made it my mission to meet a boy or man and explore his body, even though access was extremely limited.

In high school I managed to make a few new friends, but they were as sexually inexperienced as I, and so our conversations consisted of safe, artificial chatter about our favorite bands and TV shows. I tended to seek out girls who talked more than I, feeling awkward and uncomfortable with the sound of my own voice and what little I had to offer. I rarely wanted to see these girls outside of school, limiting our casual intimacies to the one-hour lunch block and quick hallway strolls between classes. Vivid delusions of social rejection, like what I'd experienced in junior high, made the idea of real intimacy far too costly. I told myself it was cooler to be an outcast anyway. I wasn't meant for the pack.

Similar to my behavior before high school, I focused vigorously on my studies, but my efforts went mostly unnoticed at school, which doubled as a convent and was set among green hills and silk floss trees. Teachers expected the very best from their students. The school's patron saint was Joan of Arc, and a life-size statue of this young, mighty woman glared at students every time we entered the library. Our skirts were measured to be just-above-the-knee length, nail polish strictly forbidden, and if you broke these rules or any others, you were issued a citation and ordered to perform some kind of tedious labor on campus. Many of the teachers were nuns, including the principal, and they made it clear that even if you thought you were doing well, you could always, *always* do better.

While I was willing to stray from perfectionism in junior high school if it meant I could be socially accepted, I now sought perfectionism as a way to secure my isolation. My studying increased significantly; I always hungered for more knowledge. I read more, taking a liking to Albert Camus, Virginia Woolf, and Joan Didion. My aversion to small talk led me to browse the school's impressive library collection during lunch for books that hadn't been assigned, educating myself on stream of consciousness and existentialism. I joined the Young Poets Society on campus, though I mostly observed the other writers and rarely shared my own work. My obsession for knowledge soon rivaled my fixation on body hair and orgasms. Intellectualism was an escape.

When I found this pressure was too much, I excused myself from class for a bathroom break. Masturbating in the school bathroom required all the usual sensations of control I'd grown used to. I had to be quiet if another girl was in the next stall. I had to keep my feet relaxed and still on the bathroom floor. And I had to be sure to achieve orgasm quickly, to avoid raising suspicions. I'd emerge from the bathroom sickened with myself but light-headed with pleasure. Were other girls doing this? I couldn't know for sure. What I did know was that they weren't talking about it in the same way that most girls didn't talk about their periods or changing bodies or anything that might've been deemed "gross" or "TMI."

I got my first period at the start of high school and considered myself a late bloomer. I based this on no evidence other than the fact that my mom had left a box of pads in my bathroom cupboard years before and I'd been dreading the day I'd have to use them. Bleeding humiliated me. I was disgusted by the sight of blood and embarrassed when I had to ask my mom to buy me more pads when I ran out. I was also paranoid that other people might be able to smell my leaky sign of womanhood and laugh at me, just like I imagined them laughing if they found out I masturbated all the time. But there was no stopping my body from what it wanted to do.

One day, in my sophomore year scripture class, we filed into the classroom to find the word *masturbation* scrawled across the green chalkboard in giant script. Giggles bubbled up from all corners of the room, while my body turned hot and tingly. Our teacher, Sister Victoria, was a petite, lighthearted woman in her sixties who seemed the only nun capable of discussing sex. She often made comments about some of the young male teachers she found handsome, which made her trustworthy to us, relatable.

When we all sat down, she stood in front of the chalkboard, a tiny figure ironically framed by a word that was far too sinful to be in such close proximity to a holy woman.

"This is an important word," she started. "Masturbation."

Snickers everywhere.

"I want you all to know that, while it's normal to become acquainted with your body, masturbation can be, well . . ." She paused. "To put it plainly, masturbation can be very dangerous."

I gulped, and the giggles subsided.

"You may find yourself staying home all day . . ."

I pictured myself in my bedroom. Feeling lonely and depressed until I stuck my hands down my pants. Then lonely and depressed all over again.

"Losing interest in your friends . . ."

What friends?

"Losing interest in your work. Losing interest in God." Her look was grave and her tone serious. It made me wonder if this had happened to Sister Victoria.

She continued her rant on the perils of masturbation. My breaths became shorter. I felt exposed, like my life was an open wound for the whole room to see, vulnerable and raw and prone to infection. As if there were a spotlight on me, or a magnifying glass. *Don't look at me*, I repeated over and over in my head. *Please, don't look at me.* Then Sister Victoria opened the floor for questions. When nobody stirred, her disposition switched to something much cheerier and so did everyone else's. We moved on to one of Jesus's many miracles, while I sat there in silence, gutted. I needed to stop, but how?

My interest in cybersex declined around this time, as its effectiveness to getting me off waned. But as my interest in cybersex went down, internet speeds were going up, a steady progression of endless resources matched with my growing habit. Although the first porn site, Sex.com, went live in 1994, streaming videos were still the stuff of dreams. Pictures were easier to find and download, and were sometimes sent via email from cybersex partners, and once in a while I found GIFs, though rarely.

Gabe's drawers never failed to make up for what the internet lacked. Finding the Tommy Lee and Pamela Anderson sex tape was one of my most exciting and equally debilitating discoveries.

It was 1998 and I was almost sixteen. The sex tape had been

passing between teenagers like precious contraband until it eventually landed in my brother's hands. I'd never had so much enticing footage at my disposal to pause or fast-forward or rewind whenever I wanted. The sex tape put me in control.

The tape was also the first porn I ever watched with another person—my brother's first serious girlfriend, Monica. It was the first time I let someone into that secret place of ecstatic moans and big, bouncing tits and massive dicks and me, the watcher, captivated by all of it. How different it was to have someone right beside me, someone just as captivated, someone to make me feel less alone. Maybe I wasn't so pathetic after all.

four

THE GIRLFRIEND

Without even knowing it, I was also becoming acquainted with meditation. I don't recall reading books on this practice, and so I'm not sure how I made the discovery, but I recognized immediately, and appreciated, how different it felt from praying, which had been full of pleading and frustration in my younger years. I picked up a CD at Ross called *Pure Moods*, a new age compilation with artists like Deep Forest and Enya, and I played this on a loop, lighting candles and incense, and settling into a feeling of deep peace. During the week, when the house was almost empty, this peace was only interrupted when Gabe fought with Monica.

Gabe started dating Monica back in high school, but now that he was enrolled in community college and juggling the possibilities for his next move, which would eventually be San Francisco, it seemed clear to everyone this move wouldn't include her. And while I didn't want them to break up, I came to crave their fights because they would often send Monica into a tantrum, after which she'd escape his bedroom for my own.

At the time, I was desperate for a real-life female role model, having long ago decided suburbia was a trap and I was meant for bigger things. Monica, three years my senior, seemed a perfect candidate.

Unlike other Mexican girls in the neighborhood, she wore dark red lipstick and had a punk-rock wardrobe—combat boots, fishnet stockings, a collection of spiked necklaces. Most girls shaved their eyebrows off and wore their boyfriend's pants and huge hoop earrings. Their idea of a fashion mag wasn't *Vogue* but *Lowrider*. She introduced me to strong female singers like Tori Amos, Johnette Napolitano, and the singer-songwriter Fiona Apple, whom I adored for her angsty lyrics.

I found the Tommy Lee and Pamela Anderson sex tape when Gabe was away from the house one day and Monica was hanging out with me. I knew it was an invasion of his privacy to go through his drawers when he wasn't around, but I'd been doing it for so long at this point, it no longer felt wrong. Monica didn't seem to mind, either.

"Maybe we'll find photos of others girls or phone numbers or something?" She seemed equally excited and afraid of the thought.

The VHS tape didn't have a label, but I knew what it was.

"I think this is porn," I said, holding up the tape. I tried not to look too excited or disinterested. I wanted her to take the lead and decide whether we should watch it.

"Yes!" she yelled, her eyes lighting up. "I know what it is! Let's watch it."

I couldn't have been happier. We giggled as we popped in the sex tape, turning the volume down to its lowest decibel so we could barely hear the moaning.

"He's superhot," Monica said. "Look how big his dick is!"

As we watched Tommy and Pam frolic around, Monica's giggling softened and mine became shrill and frantic. I felt uncomfortable watching the tape with her because I was getting turned on, and I couldn't just excuse myself for relief, nor could I ask her questions about sex because she was my brother's girlfriend; I didn't want mental images of the two of them in my head.

When my feelings got unbearable so that I had to look down to keep from soaking through my pants, Monica said, abruptly, "You know, if you were a man, I'd choose you over your brother." The words shot through my body like an electric surge. I didn't know what to say, and so I giggled more, my legs feeling like rubber beneath me, my stomach aching with desire.

That night, Monica slept over, even though she and my brother were still fighting as usual. My parents' house rules forbade the two of them from sleeping in my brother's bed, and so she slept in my bed, which had happened before. Only this night felt different. This night I felt too excited to be sleepy.

We lay there in the dark for a while, our bodies pushed together in the twin-size bed, my back to her stomach.

"Turn around," she finally whispered, saving me from the racing fantasies in my head, for which I had not yet found relief—Tommy's dick, Pam's tits, the two of us sharing that erotic moment together.

I rolled my body around and faced her, though I could barely make out her big green eyes.

"Hi," she said.

Before I could say hi back, though I may not have said anything, as I seemed to have lost my voice, she leaned in and softly kissed me on the mouth with her full lips. My first kiss.

I froze.

"Kiss me back," she said, pulling her face away from mine. She sounded annoyed.

That's when I found my voice and said something I have been humiliated and equally confused about ever since.

"Not today, Junior!" I shot back, giggling again. Then I flipped my body back around so I wasn't facing her anymore.

I'm pretty sure I was referencing a line in *Billy Madison*, when Adam Sandler's jackass character hassles a boy who has trouble reading aloud, by shouting, "T-t-today, Junior!" but why I would feel the need to reference an Adam Sandler movie at that sensual moment is still a mystery.

I buried my face in the sheets, Monica fell asleep, and she and my brother ultimately broke up just like everyone knew they would.

◆

As awkward as that moment had been with Monica, I convinced myself that this awkwardness had everything to do with the fact that she was not just my brother's girlfriend but also a girl. And even though my sexual attraction to other girls was obvious, I was no lesbian.

Growing up, I never heard anyone berate homosexuality or, in my case, bisexuality, but I never heard anyone praise these orientations either. The only time I remember my parents addressing the topic was when they talked about my dad's cousin Rafa, a gay man who had been robbed and murdered on the streets of Mexico City.

Because I had such little context for these complex feelings, when same-sex sexual arousal came up for me, I discovered another source of shame. Yet the more I tried to suppress this longing, the more I could not. My hunger for women followed me around constantly, and I was always scared of being found out. This led me to further distance myself from other girls and feel stressed in the most ordinary of situations, never holding eye contact too long, pulling away from hugs, declining phone calls and social invitations. I turned my attention to men, reminding myself like one of those Catholic counselors who make it their mission to cure gayness: *Liking men is normal. Don't be weird.* I told myself that had I been in bed with a guy that night instead of Monica, he would have known how to keep me from freaking out. He would have known how to crack me open and pull away the weirdness to reveal the vixen that lived within.

At least that's what I hoped.

I became preoccupied with finding "the one," clinging to the idea that satisfaction lived outside of me. I was confident I would visit exotic places and manifest artistic fame and intellectual excellence in adulthood, but I didn't want to wait until adulthood to feel real human affection. And the only human affection I was after was in the form of heterosexual sex. I fantasized about when and how I would lose my virginity and become a woman of the world, and I imagined that once I had sex, I would lose interest in my fixations. Sex would be the mother of all accomplishments.

But first I needed to find a boy. Or be found by one.

◆

I was sixteen when I met Vincent, the mocha-skinned nephew of my mom's friend. Tall, athletic, and proudly Latino, Vincent played high school football, listened to rap music, and lived an hour away from us. On the weekends, we saw action-packed movies he picked and took long drives during which I let him do most of the talking, playing the polite, observant girl I mastered with all my friends at school. He covered everything from football to baseball to hockey to weightlifting to how funny and cool his friends were. I smiled enthusiastically and acted interested.

Having a weekend boyfriend was an ideal scenario for me. Monday through Thursday, I obsessed about what we would do on the upcoming weekend, sometimes unable to sleep from excitement. On Fridays, before seeing him, I locked myself in my bathroom, stripped down to nakedness and did a lengthy examination to ensure that my body was flawless, making sure I had removed every last hair from my arms, legs, upper lip, knuckles, everywhere. All week I had imagined our safe conversation transitioning into making out and then turning into sex shortly thereafter, but I was simultaneously filled with dread because I had no idea how any of this worked in real life. I had seen enough porn to think I knew, but trying these things I watched seemed infinitely more intimidating.

This neurotic examination of my body became standard practice whenever I was romantically involved after Vincent. Whether I was into the guy or not, I put myself to work because I figured that's what women did. I'd set up shop and primp and pick in the bathroom to emerge a better me.

But that's not all. Over time, my fixation with hair removal became a compulsion not unlike masturbation. Even when I wasn't dating anyone, I came to rely on various habits designed to whisk hours away in bulk while I achieved temporary perfection. Removing all my hair was obviously futile, and thus maddening, but I came to crave the sting of a tweezers' pluck and the soapy sweep of a razor against flesh. I got hooked on nail salons, which were aplenty in my neighborhood. Every two weeks I'd entrust thin, jade-wearing Vietnamese women not only with the upkeep of my cuticles but also with the maintenance of my eyebrows, upper lip, sideburns, and anywhere else I noticed unsightliness rising from my skin.[8]

---

8   The author and activist Naomi Wolf would say I was caught up in "the beauty myth." This unhealthy obsession with physical perfection traps the modern woman in a never-ending spiral of self-consciousness and self-hatred as she attempts to fulfill society's impossible standards of flawless beauty. Wolf writes in *The Beauty Myth*, "As women released themselves from the feminine mystique of domesticity, the beauty myth took over its lost ground, expanding as it waned to carry on its work of social control."

Vincent and I were completely incompatible, but he was interested enough to hang out with me, so I figured he was probably interested enough to have sex with me. That was all that mattered. Another chance might not roll around again.

Our first make-out session was awkward and clumsy. It happened during our third weekend together, when we found ourselves conveniently alone at my house. After browsing the VHS tapes, Vincent found a *Football Follies* yawner and popped it in. Three minutes later, minutes we spent pretending to watch the tape, he tackled my face with his open mouth and darting tongue, and while I tried my best to keep my eyes closed and refrain from laughing, our teeth crashed and collided. When we stopped to look at each other or talk, our words spilled out sloppy and senseless. So to avoid the talk (or lack thereof) we continued with this uncomfortable kissing until the moment when, in finally exploring one of my arms with his wobbly hands, Vincent stopped kissing and looked down. I did too.

"Do you shave your arms?" He was rubbing near my elbow, where I saw about eight or nine short, black, thick hairs in a rectangular patch.

"No," I lied. I leaned in to kiss him again, but he kept rubbing. I felt my face heating up and knew I would be blushing in no time—then he would know, my face would be proof. He'd know that underneath my beautiful, hairless arms were apelike, monstrous things, that I was a beast in disguise. So I did what I had to—the one thing that I knew would distract him. I grabbed his hand and shoved it under my blouse. Somehow, the only way to mask my insecurity was to overpower it with sex.

We lay down and he closed his eyes again while he fondled my breasts over my cotton bra, his erection undeniably present against my jeans. And while I wanted to reach for his penis, to have one finally inside me, I found myself scared and motionless. I wasn't even sure I was good at kissing, so what if I was just as terrible at sex?

We didn't have sex that day, or any other day during the next couple of months we spent our weekends together. He didn't seem eager to explore anything beyond second base, and I took this unwillingness as certain rejection and didn't push it. In all the movies I'd ever watched, men were the ones who made the first move. Women, it seemed, either played hard to get and were labeled dick-teasing prudes, or they quickly gave in and were called sluts and whores. I wasn't sure which was better to be, but I knew that my desire was becoming unbearably urgent.

◆

Like the books and late-night videos I feasted on, fashion magazines also became an obsession, their covers offering new and beautiful white actresses I tried to emulate as best I could. Gwyneth Paltrow playing Estella in the adaptation of *Great Expectations* became my ideal of beauty, appearing smooth and slim and seductive throughout the film. I coveted her ability to drive Finn crazy and simultaneously hold his desire over decades, and thought to myself, *This is power.* I copied dramatic gazes from perfume ads, refused to leave the house without red lipstick, bought green contact lenses to cover up my brown hue, used hair serums, and coated my face in my mom's expensive facial creams that smelled like jasmine and perfection. They were a godsend; I could always count on my mom's drawers for a variety of transformative beauty products whenever I was feeling ugly.

Though my mom often said I was beautiful and tried to boost my ego whenever possible, she wasn't very successful at masking her own insecurities.

"*Mija*," she'd say, whenever I'd stumble upon her in the bath-room, her curling iron hot, her makeup spread across the coun-tertops like animal-tested confetti. "Tell me if I look OK." Her face would be twisted and a little afraid, expecting the worst. I'd tell her she looked great, and she always did, but it didn't matter. "You're only saying that because you love me. But thanks."

No matter how hard she tried to find peace with her body, there always seemed to be more my mom could do.[9] She had tried numerous diet fads, experimented with eyelash extensions, paid big bucks for Botox, and always made it clear a facelift was in her future. For her, beauty products and designer labels were key to fitting in. Women were supposed to keep up and keep it together, or else you became fodder for the cruelest gossip. You wouldn't find gray in my mom's hair, a makeup product other than Chanel in her vanity drawers, and her nails were always long and immacu-lately shaped.

Like my mom, I was adamant about hiding this insecurity from others. Which is why this self-hating, back-braced little girl was able to muster the courage to enter the Miss Montebello Beauty Pageant.

My mom was the one who first showed me the ad for the pag-eant, and my initial reaction was terror.

"You can't be serious," I told her, holding back the laughter.

---

9   Dr. Leslie Sim, clinical director of Mayo Clinic's eating-disorders pro-gram and a child psychologist, reported to *USA Today*, "Moms are probably the most important influence on a daughter's body image. Even if a mom says to the daughter, 'You look so beautiful, but I'm so fat,' it can be detrimental." Research has shown the less emphasis a mother puts on outward appearance, either criticizing or complimenting herself, her daughter, and others, the more likely her daughter will have high self-esteem.

Beauty pageants were for the kinds of girls who wore high heels, looked fabulous in bikinis, dated the quarterback.

"You might have fun!" she insisted. "Plus, there's free clothes, trips, money . . ." She listed all the highlights of the pageant, but not the obvious negatives. Still, one thought caught my attention: trips.

"What do I have to do for that stuff though?" I asked. "Walk around in a bathing suit? Because, I promise you, I won't do that." I put the newspaper down on the kitchen table.

"Who knows, maybe there's no bathing suit. Just think about it, OK?" Though my mom didn't verbally push the topic after that, she did cut the ad from the newspaper and post it to the fridge. So every time I went to get a snack throughout the next week, there, accompanying my hunger, was the ad.

The more I saw the ad and the more I thought about the pageant, the more I craved the challenge. I knew that if I won, I'd have something concrete to prove I'd transcended my awkward younger years. The fact was that I wanted to believe total transformation was possible. I wanted to be done with the uncertainty of whether I was desirable. A crown would be the ideal confirmation.

I showed up at the first meeting with other Mexican girls who wore lots of makeup, short skirts, and glares that said not to fuck with them. These girls were not like the kind I hung out with at school. They were well put together and full of sass. And they were my competition. I needed to beat them, not befriend them.

Dressed up as a "scholarship competition," the pageant was not traditional; there'd be no parading around in swimsuits or answering impromptu questions by hunks like Mario Lopez. The pageant coordinator, a corporate-looking Mexican woman with blond highlights and perfectly arched eyebrows, told us there would be fashion shows at our local mall, appearances in nearby city parades, speech writing, and lots of hair, makeup, and etiquette training. Plus, we'd have bonding time with the other girls, building friendships that would last a lifetime.

My mom, who had become increasingly concerned about my lack of friends, was convinced that I had been cured of my social awkwardness merely for agreeing to compete. I told her I only wanted the prizes and money and trips that were promised for every contestant, even those who didn't win. Secretly I obsessed about the gratifying title and how this title would transform me. Despite her hopeful boasts to everyone that I was making new friends with the other contestants, I was often off in the corner alone, hoping my silence gave me an air of mystery.

Though I knew the pageant would involve public speaking, I somehow considered that less threatening than normal, day-to-day conversation, reassuring myself that the people in the crowd would never actually know the real me. They'd get some pretty words in nice packaging and a big fake smile. There was no room to be especially vulnerable.

Over the months of preparation for the pageant, all the contestants were treated to luncheons, where we were meant to mingle but I stuck to the platters of chopped-up vegetables with lite ranch and endless trays of fruit. We were armed with a variety of different outfits, from business suits to ball gowns, and I found out that pageant girls actually do use Vaseline on their teeth to sustain fake smiling with minimal effort. Simply slather the gooey gunk all over your teeth and gums, it turns out, and your face muscles are relieved.

I considered dropping out of the pageant several times at the terror of being scrutinized by a panel of judges. But always I convinced myself to hold out for the pageant and cash prizes like I said I would. I didn't want to look like a failure. Especially to all the other girls I deemed unworthy.

A few days before the pageant, we were all sitting around a large table at Denny's, ordering salads without dressing—the menu clearly favored burgers and milk shakes. We were playing the part of soft-spoken, healthy-eating, perfect pageant girls when one pretty girl interrupted the act. Andy was, by far, the prettiest and most perfect-looking. I detested her.

"I forgot to shave today! I can't believe it! I've been so busy with rehearsing, it totally slipped my mind!" She was hysterical, staring down at her prickly arms in disgust. I guess I'd been so busy with my own rehearsing that I'd missed her flaw.

"Oh yeah!" Another girl sitting a few seats to her right leaned over and examined the pretty girl's arms. Then she flung out her own arm for inspection. It was clean and smooth and she was proud of it.

One by one, every girl at the table, except myself, offered her arm for comparison. I was shocked and relieved all at once. One girl confessed that while sometimes she forgot to shave her legs, she always remembered her arms. Another confided that she'd tried burning her hair once and that gave her the best results—some of the hair had never grown back. I sat there amused, listening to them, relating to them. We were all in the same boat, trying our hardest to live a lie. Instead of embracing them as comrades, I reacted with domination. Why not let them think I was naturally flawless? That I was, in fact, perfect, exactly like they hoped to be?

I didn't know then, not entirely, what a nasty game I was learning to play. I already had trouble connecting with other girls and women, yet the pageant would make connection even more unfavorable. The need to feel superior to other women would frequently turn into feeling less than other women, but once I was caught up in the currents of this painful pastime, it was impossible to escape.

On the day of the pageant, each of the contestants had to privately face the panel of judges before the actual public event. We were told there would be a series of questions, but there were no details on what these questions could be. I wore one of the corporate outfits I'd been given—a gray, knee-length dress and nude nylons—and sat before the eight serious judges in complete trepidation.

"Tell us about yourself," one of the female judges began. She wore a dark blazer and a pencil skirt, black nylons and a necklace of pearls, and her request may have sounded simple, but for me, it was far too complex. What could I possibly say?

"I'm Erica. I'm seventeen." I gulped the air. "And I'm a writer."

I had never made a declaration like that, and I surprised myself by saying it.

"A writer?" Another judge spoke up. "What do you write?"

"I write about myself," I said. "About how things are. About what I want to do and who I want to be." *Please change the subject*, I thought to myself. *Ask me what I'd do with a million dollars; maybe I could answer that. Ask me about world peace.*

"And what do you want to do?" One of the younger judges, a blond guy with crystal-blue eyes, smiled when he spoke.

"I want to see places," I answered, my face already becoming hot and palms wet. "I want to live in France, learn foreign languages, maybe learn to paint, possibly become a teacher . . ." I went off in tangents, describing the exotic endeavors I'd spent years collecting. And the more I spoke, the easier the answers rolled out of me. Soon the interview was over.

When the time came for the actual pageant, I walked the stage with perfect posture, not from balancing books on my head but because the metal rods in my back gave me no other choice. The room was mostly dark, with bright spotlights pointed at the stage, and so, luckily, I didn't have to make eye contact with anyone in the crowd. During the talent portion of the pageant, some girls sang and others danced. I emerged with a camera, dressed like a beatnik, and pretended to take photos of the crowd to show that I was an artist.

When it was time for the speech, each of the girls offered her story—the obstacles she'd faced and the dreams that she sought. I wore a gleaming red gown that matched my red lips and rattled off my perfectly memorized speech about the hardships of having to leave school and all my "friends" because of the surgery that had nearly killed me—an embellishment I figured would win me some pity points. My closing line was taken from a book of inspirational quotes and really had nothing to do with the speech I'd thrown at the crowd.

" 'You make a living by what you get,' " I said, taking a dramatic pause. " 'You make a life by what you give.' " I liked the sentiment of the quote and its clever play on words, but I knew it was bullshit coming out of my mouth. What could I possibly give to anyone? A tutorial on how to find the best porn? How to keep their bodies in tip-top, hairless shape? How to make it through high school without making any real friends? I felt like a fraud, but I didn't care. All that mattered was winning.

After the last girl had given her speech, the judges handed in their points to be tallied in a fifteen-minute interlude of suspense. Then the previous Miss Montebello, a skinny girl with long dark hair and fake nails, took to the stage to give her last walk as queen. She smiled and waved to the audience and then made her way to the microphone to announce the winner. All of us girls were at the back of the stage, lined up in our shimmery dresses, our Vaseline-enforced smiles beaming at the faceless crowd. I felt confident with how things had played out, but I was still worried. I went over the pageant in my head to see if there was anything I could have improved. I had answered all the questions in the interview, I hadn't forgotten any of my lines, I hadn't fallen in my heels, my lipstick was intact . . .

"Erica!" the girl next to me nudged me and I snapped out of my trance as ex–Miss Montebello balanced the heavy crown on my head, forcing me to put in extra effort to keep my chin raised and face forward despite the weight. Then she placed a sash over my body and draped a big red robe over my shoulders so that I could barely take a step.

The crowd cheered and whistled, and I had to make my way to the front of the stage, my petite body trudging under the heavy indicators of my most delicious triumph. The flashing of cameras showered over me and I smiled wide, laughing in self-satisfaction.

The title gave me a boost of confidence I had never before experienced. Just like those attractive guests on *Montel* or *Maury* who used daytime TV to confront their childhood bullies and flaunt their newfound good looks, I, too, was a success story. And all the secret effort I put into my body—the long hours I'd sacrificed pursuing perfection—had brought me to this point. I knew then that I'd have to keep up my hard work if the result was the recognition of others and feeling like someone of value. I made a promise to myself to always be this way.

◆

The surge of empowerment didn't last long. I still found myself uncomfortable around people and had no hope for effortless beauty.

My beauty took work. But as I grew up a little, I also seemed to grow more appealing to the opposite sex. When I caught a man checking me out, I felt a rush of validation course through me, a physical sensation that was almost as intense as when I sought out porn clips.

The internet was becoming more enticing as the technology grew more sophisticated. Speeds went up in what felt like a daily progression and, soon enough, streaming porn sites popped up across the vast digital underworld. When my parents bought me a laptop, I found it even harder to leave my room.

The more I viewed porn, the more anxiety I had about being caught.[10] To calm the panic, I took my laptop into the closet and pleasured myself in there—my body crammed between my clothes and books. I also feared the smell of my secret stayed on my fingers and that no matter how hard I scrubbed, the shaming stench trapped under my nails and embedded in the fine creases that make up my fingerprints would give me away. I imagined people around me whispering among themselves. I imagined old, wrinkled women who made it to the end of their days without having ever fallen into my bad ways, shaking their heads, muttering to themselves, "When will it ever be enough?"

The type of porn I watched varied from day to day. My young lust gravitated to categories like cheerleaders, schoolgirls, and teens,

---

10   In a 2011 article for *The Guardian* called "Why More and More Women Are Using Pornography," UK porn counselor Jason Dean cited one in three clients seeking help for porn addiction were women. The main contrast between his male and female clients? Guilt. "Porn addiction is seen as a man's problem—and therefore not acceptable for women," said Dean. "There's a real sense among women that it's bad, dirty, wrong, and they're often unable to get beyond that."

probably because I related to the youthful theme. I was also drawn to lesbian scenes, which were equally exciting regardless of the age of the actresses. While masturbating had been a daily habit for years, porn had been an occasional treat—but that was about to change.[11]

When I did pry myself out of the house, I carried the scenes around with me all day, fantasizing about the people around me and imagining what we'd do if given a dark room and opportunity. And as exciting as it was to feel a man's eyes on me, when it didn't happen, I felt empty and pathetic.

Because I went to a same-sex school, finding a man to squash my virginity like the disgusting pest it was to me would require having to be social and meet one. So I stepped outside my box, as uncomfortable as it was, and went out more with girls from school in hopes that their normalcy would lead me to a penis.

With social anxiety as severe as mine, a normal, everyday conversation could be torture. Panic surrounded simple situations like shared dinners and lunches, birthday parties and car rides. Even standing in line at Starbucks would be excruciating if small talk got thrown into the mix. But I was willing to subject myself to this discomfort if it meant meeting a guy.

◆

Sometime in the middle of my senior year, I met Alex. I was at a restaurant with some girls from school. He was strong in the

---

11   A study by the University of New Hampshire in 2006 found that 93 percent of boys and 62 percent of girls were exposed to online pornography during their adolescence, and the National Coalition for the Protection of Children & Families reported in 2010 that 47 percent of US families claimed that pornography was a problem in their home.

shoulders and had deep-blue eyes. When I caught him staring at me over the tables, I felt the room fall away, the clatter of plates and cutlery drowned out by the electricity of being looked at like that. I held his gaze, feeling terrified but driven.

"I have to know the name of such a beautiful woman," he said, when he approached our table. This seemed a joke; I'd never been called a woman before and certainly didn't feel like one. He sat down next to me, ordered a coffee, and asked me questions about myself. I was nervous, and he could tell, so he placed his hand on my knee, a thrilling sensation.

Days later, on our first date, Alex—who'd been born in Mexico City but looked white—picked me up from my parents' house in his red Mustang convertible. He was charming and confident, asking them thoughtful questions about my dad's work and commenting on the architecture of our house. I could tell by the way my mom looked at him and then at me, approvingly, that she, too, was impressed.

He drove us to Griffith Park, where he put a blanket down on warm grass and fed me strawberries while Billie Holiday crooned from his car speakers. He told me he played the saxophone, and talked about jazz music being "beautiful and chaotic," like life. He was studying architecture and carpentry, he said, and was always building something. Then he showed me his hands. I studied them with their rough calluses and scars, and when he cradled my head in these hands as he kissed me, I felt something I had never felt before. It was as if I had risen out of my body and could see myself from some separate, otherworldly place. I hoped this feeling was love.

Alex was not that much older, but he was wise and witty and had a broad knowledge about literature, art, music, and other cultures, making the three years between us feel like decades. He took me to nice restaurants with live music and LA's best beaches and hotspots, as if I were a tourist. But soon the places became more secluded, and making out always led to us getting undressed. Just before he'd remove his boxer briefs, I'd stop him and ask if he had a condom.

"No, I don't like the way they feel. But don't worry, I don't have any diseases."

Although I should have been worried about diseases, I would be lying if I said that that was my primary concern. My mom had been looking down on teenage mothers for as far back as I could remember and I knew I couldn't become one. It also hadn't crossed my mind that girls could buy condoms too.

I hadn't the slightest clue how to please a man, and I was terrified of embarrassing myself with Alex. I liked him too much. What if he thought I was terrible and left me? I clung to the power that I saw in Estella from *Great Expectations*, how she continued to hold Finn's interest in denying him. But refusing Alex only agitated him. And agitation turned to obsession. No longer did we go to beaches and parks or even restaurants; instead, he'd pick me up and drive me straight to parking garages or empty lots by abandoned buildings and train tracks and pounce on me in the backseat.

Still, he never brought a condom. All these years later, I have trouble figuring out why he wouldn't just give in and wear one, because I probably would've slept with him if he had. I think it always came back to the fact that he needed to have it his way. This was his particular thrill. And he struck me as the kind of man who was rarely denied.

When I told him, repeatedly, that I wasn't ready to have sex with him without a condom, he'd laugh at me, saying that I was a little girl, a "tease," and that I was wasting his time for my own pleasure. He'd reminisce, openly, about ex-lovers and then tell me that, actually, they weren't ex-lovers—he was fucking lots of women, older and experienced women.

"That's why I only see you on weekends," he said. "I'm busy with real women during the week."

He told me this and I began to hate him as much as I felt I loved him, equating my emotions with his description of jazz music, beautiful and chaotic. Yet I continued to answer his phone calls and let him take me to the dark empty places where he'd try and fail again and again. All along, I held tight to the idea that somehow he would revert to who he was in the beginning: romantic, inspiring, respectful.

The last "date" we had was just a few days after Christmas. I bought him a two-disc jazz compilation from Tower Records and wrapped it in festive red-and-green tissue paper, tied neatly with a gold bow. It was late, and we were parked up on a hill not far from my house where he read the musicians' names off the compilation box, looking bored and unimpressed. He sighed and thanked me, apologizing for not getting me a gift, though the apology did not feel genuine. We didn't say anything for a few minutes as he popped one of the CDs into his car's disc player and we sat there immersed in the noise.

Feeling nauseated with myself for not being able to please him, I whispered, "I think I'm ready."

He didn't look at me. "Ready for what?"

I reached my shaky, sweaty hand over across the seat and placed it on his crotch, unaware of what to do next. He didn't make any moves, and so I rubbed gently, up and down, up and

down, hoping he'd give some sort of instruction. I felt him growing through his jeans, but he only sighed impatiently. I unzipped
him and paused.

"Well?" he said.

I didn't say anything. I just stared. That's when he took my
head in his hardworking hands and pushed me down. I instinc-
tively hesitated, jerking back, wanting to tell him I wasn't ready
after all, but he just said, "Open your mouth," and I complied.

It didn't take long for me to realize that I did, in fact, know how
to please a man. I successfully satisfied him in a few minutes and
he used the red-and-green tissue paper to clean himself. After he'd
zipped up his pants and thanked me, he dropped me off at my
house, and I didn't hear from him again.

◆

I got my first job a few months before high school was over, waitressing at a local diner. I was good at it—balancing multiple plates
in my arms and pouring coffee without spilling a drip. But it was
a shitty restaurant. There were gnats in the blue cheese and they
served leftover dinner rolls from the night before. A family of cock-
roaches lived in the storage room. Some of the waitresses were
sleeping with the Armenian owner, a short, graying, unattractive
man in his late fifties. This made me feel awkward every time he
called me over to his office to give me the week's schedule or hand
me the credit card tips in cash, telling me to smile more, that I was
so much prettier when I smiled.

Roberto was a mechanic from Jalisco, Mexico, who often left
me big tips. He'd come in, ask for coffee, and I'd watch his dirty
hands, his fingernails black from oil and dirt and debris. He'd
pick up and drink, set it down and sigh, pick it up and drink,
set it down and sigh. I only worked at that restaurant for three

months, and for three months, he always requested to sit in my section.

He was not the kind of person who typically interested me, and he was much older than I was, at least a decade. This worried my parents, especially my dad, who seemed suspicious when Roberto started coming around to pick me up and take me out, but they never forbade it. I think they were just happy I was getting out of my room. Our conversations were simple, since Roberto hardly spoke English and I only knew a handful of Spanish words, and he hadn't finished school, making him entirely different from Alex. This disparity comforted me. Roberto felt safer in comparison. He'd drive me to Santa Monica and Malibu, where I'd dip my toes in the water and he'd tell me stories about Mexico. We'd eat at a variety of colorful Mexican restaurants, where he'd tease me for not knowing all the food items, calling me a *gringa*, a whitey.

I lost my virginity to him on what was supposed to be a trip to Disneyland, though we didn't make it all the way there. Instead, we pulled over at the Angel Inn in Anaheim and I let him fuck me without a condom because, like Alex, he said he didn't have one, but unlike my old self, I didn't care anymore. I was too lazy to go through that whole game again, and I didn't want to feel that sting of rejection I had when a mere blow job hadn't kept Alex around. What Alex wanted was for me to concede. I understood that now. And I was ready to be a girl who conceded. Who didn't give a fuck. Who was wild and careless and sexual and grown-up.

The room smelled of lingering sweat and cigarettes, and I remember the scratching of his white socks against my ankles and how I wished he'd been barefoot. I stared at his chest the whole way through, the name *Marisela* scrawled across in faded black ink, the proof that at least one other person had been there first.

He came inside me and I didn't even come close, and afterward, he held me tight in his hairy arms, calling me his little princess, telling me he'd take care of me forever.

We continued sleeping together through the end of high school, and I found a sense of power in being able to confess to girls at school that I had traversed into the nonvirginal life. I thought to myself that maybe this was all I needed to connect with others, because small talk suddenly seemed easier. In retrospect, I wasn't really connecting, because hardly any of the girls I knew were having sex yet. Instead, I preached. And I loved saying that I didn't use condoms; it made me feel dangerous.

"But what if you get pregnant?" one of them asked.

I shrugged. "Abortion, I guess. Or have it—I don't know. Whatever he wants." I was clueless, actually, but completely malleable. I meant what I said to the girls in that I was willing to take on whatever life decision Roberto made for us so long as he kept sticking his dick inside me and keeping me from the isolation of my bedroom. To me, his presence confirmed that I was worthy of someone else's desire, that I might not always be alone and unlovable.

While I was happy to be having sex in various backseats and the motel rooms Roberto rented by the hour, I was irked that I never had an orgasm during sex. I had been giving myself enough orgasms to know how to get there, and I watched enough porn to know that he seemed to be trying, but it never happened. When I worked up the courage to ask him about it one night after he'd finished, he just laughed. "Next time," he said, and then he kissed me on the forehead and got dressed.

Luckily I didn't get pregnant all those times we had unprotected sex, but he seemed disappointed about this. He often told me he was ready to have a kid, and as soon as I was older (which meant legal), we'd get married and start building our little family. And while the lack of orgasms worried me, I didn't think, not even once, that it was anything he was doing wrong as a lover. I was sure that all that time I had spent with my hands in my pants had ruined me for real sex. There was something new to be ashamed about.

◆

It was the summer after high school and I was working at another restaurant, one that paid me more, when a pretty girl with big green eyes sat down and asked for pancakes. When I brought them to her, she smiled and said, "You're Erica?"

"Yes," I answered. "How did you know?"

She pointed at my name tag and smiled. "Oh, yeah." I smiled back.

"You're beautiful," she said, which made me blush.

I took care of my other customers, but I could feel her eyes on me the whole time, which made me feel clumsy yet flattered.

When she left the restaurant, she left behind a long note. When I saw it, I felt giddy, thinking she had penned me a love letter. Instead, the note detailed how Roberto had been playing us both for the past few months. She had known for a while and she was sorry to just be telling me now, but she was in love with him and she wasn't going away. In the note, she said she felt sorry for me, being as young as I was, although she hadn't looked much older.

I was crushed. But my answer was to keep seeing Roberto for a few more months, and in between heated arguments, where he'd deny everything and then confess to loving us both, we'd have frantic make-up sex and I'd try and try and try to get pregnant and make him mine.

"The oldest trick in the book," my mom used to say about women who did this sort of thing. "And it never ends well."

I didn't get pregnant, but I did pick up a new notion: men were selfish pricks. And the only way to prevent one from stealing my dignity again was to break him before he had a chance to break me.

five

THE MEAN GIRL

"We're not making love," I whispered into his ear. "We're fucking."

About six months had passed since I ended things with Roberto and I was already trying to claw my way out of another relationship. Jarrod was sensitive and serious, and I quickly learned how easy it was to hurt him.

When we started going out, I was enrolled in community college in Pasadena, right at the beginning of the early 2000s, taking the required classes in English and the humanities but still living at my parents' house to save money. I despised living under their watchful eyes, but at least I had my own car—a convertible Mustang they bought for me just after finishing high school. I'd often take long drives to the beach—Malibu, Santa Monica, and Venice, sacred destinations, where I parked by the water and scribbled down my thoughts before driving home again.

I had bumped into Jarrod at the city hall, where I was making an appearance as Miss Montebello and he was requesting funding for a skateboarding park. It had been a few years since I'd seen him flying past on his skateboard, a tall boy with scrapes on his knees and bloodshot eyes from smoking weed all day. He was an adult now, serious and handsome and involved in his community. In the past, running into someone attractive would've sent me into an awkward spiral, avoiding eye contact and scurrying away to the safety of my personal space. But not anymore. Now I felt capable of approaching a man I desired and saying hello.

With Jarrod, I was not as meek as I usually was around people, despite the attraction. Conversation was easy, and I was drawn to his ideas and willing to share my own, as silly as they sometimes sounded in my head. I loved hearing him talk about Picasso's Blue Period and the politics of street art. And he seemed genuinely interested in me, not just my body, but deeper—the things I cared about, the books I was reading, and all the things I wanted to do with my life. He even wanted to read my writing, and I surprised myself when I allowed it. I shared some of my most private thoughts on those pages, about how Alex and Roberto had treated me poorly and how terrible I felt about myself in the aftermath. When he called me up to tell me what he thought, he didn't offer me pity like I thought he would. He told me I had a gift.

Although we'd been going out for only a few months, Jarrod and I had known each other for years. We attended the same elementary school, and our parents were old friends, but because we were two years apart, our interactions were brief and limited.

Like me, Jarrod was often picked on by classmates, only his oddity wasn't a back brace but a nervous habit of sucking on his fingers. Unlike me, instead of being bullied into submission, he was aggressive and fought back. He grew strong and tall when he hit puberty, and most of the girls at school fawned over his good looks and how masterful he was on his skateboard. His talent would later earn him the attention of skate brands and a bit of money, which he mostly spent on art supplies and pot.

When we had sex for the first time in the front seat of his silver Nissan Sentra, I remember the change that came over him. It was like I had cast a spell with my vagina and suddenly he was mine. Completely, sincerely mine. Now, everywhere I looked there he was—waiting for me outside my lecture hall, sitting on the hood of my car, on the front steps to my house. He wrote me passionate love poems and left them in my drawers so I wouldn't find them until days or weeks later. Or sometimes he'd leave them on the windshield of my car when it was parked in one of the crowded lots on campus. I never knew how he found my car in those parking lots. The task must have taken him hours each time, but he was determined to make grand gestures with his love, calling me multiple times a day to tell me he missed me, he was thinking of me, he loved me.

I had never experienced this kind of adulation before, but I ran with it as hard and as fast as I could. His devotion both amused and invigorated me. He was always willing to satisfy any of my requests, and I had no reservations about making new ones all the time. "Fuck me again." Done. "Buy me a piece of jewelry." Done. "Get a tattoo of my star sign." Done. And if he even hinted at hesitation to one of my requests, I'd put my hands down his pants or detach completely so he'd think I'd never put my hands down his pants again. I always got my way.

I also figured out how to have an orgasm during sex. I could masturbate with him inside me, something that hadn't occurred to me with Roberto. It's not that I never saw porn stars masturbate while having sex; I'd simply been too shy to do it myself. I was better at the required moaning and mimicking Roberto's satisfaction after he'd finished. With Jarrod, I felt comfortable enough that I didn't need to pretend, and it made sex all the more enjoyable.

Another new venture was trying pot. I smoked with Jarrod

twice, and both times made me paranoid. Everything I said or thought while high seemed either too profound or nonsensical, and I couldn't handle these extremes. I preferred the alcohol he stole from his parents' cabinets, and later, the random pills he stored in unlabeled prescription bottles. I wasn't sure what these pills were—and I didn't ask—but I liked how they made me feel: numb. And I came to crave this numbness while I lounged on his bed, watching him make paintings on the other side of his room. When the booze and pills wore off, I'd take off my clothes and call him back to the bed.

But when we weren't having sex or getting fucked up, I got bored. And the boredom would invariably morph into anger. Although I found him handsome and interesting and I felt adored and powerful in his presence, there was something missing. The idea of freedom kept creeping into my mind.

One day, a few months into dating, I saw my way out: his stories. I'd noticed that many of his elaborate tales had too many holes in them to be true. Like skateboarding across every European country, or the time he once let a cabdriver take him from California to New York.

"How did you have money for a trip like that?" I asked, rolling my eyes as I looked away.

"I broke into an ATM machine and took off with a bag of cash," he said, as if the answer were obvious.

But I, too, would be lying if I said that his dishonesty upset me. I was relieved. His lying meant that I could exit the relationship and still be the good guy. He could be the one at fault and I could be the kind of person who held integrity in the highest regard. It was so much easier than telling the truth: I needed drama; I needed him to be a prick. I wanted to feel something Jarrod couldn't give me.

So I ended things, at Duke's restaurant in Malibu, just off the Pacific Coast Highway. Biting into a piece of medium-rare filet mignon, I glanced over at the obscure expanse of the ocean and then back at him and said, "It's not you. It's me." Then I laughed at how that sounded. "Isn't that what people say?" I'd never broken up with a person before. This was new territory.

He didn't reply or touch his food. He just stared down at his plate while I talked and laughed and ate the expensive meal I wouldn't be buying. But his silence annoyed me, and annoyance quickly turned to anger. I wanted him to put up a fight or beg me to change my mind, not just sit there and take it.

Only later, after he'd driven us back to his house and I'd climbed on top of him did he finally react the way I wanted him to. I waited until he came, his body spasming beneath my own, and then I climbed off abruptly, pushing his arms away when he tried to keep me close. That's when he started weeping, first softly, and then progressively louder, curling his muscular body into a ball on his bedsheets. He looked like a child instead of the six-foot-three man that he was. I sighed, turning away to focus on a painting on the other side of his bedroom—a red-and-purple face of a monster, which he'd partly painted with his own blood. Seeing him naked and sobbing into his sheets, I felt guilty but utterly satisfied. Vicious but adored. When he quieted down, I gathered up my things and asked him to drive me home. But pulling away only sent him into overdrive. He continued showing up unannounced at my house or on campus, with buckets full of red roses, longer poems, and more pills. I felt suffocated, but I would only muster the courage to stay away from him after I'd lined up his replacement.

I knew I wouldn't find a new boyfriend on campus. I'd been like a ghost there, doing well in the few classes I was taking but not making an effort to build friendships or scope out any guys. So I decided to stick with what I knew. I picked up my phone and dialed a number I hadn't dialed in over a year. Alex. The kind of guy who considered an empty parking lot an appropriate date destination. The kind of guy who didn't call you back once he came in your mouth.

Dialing his number, I thought I might throw up from nervousness. I was hot and tingly, my adrenaline racing, my throat clenched. I tried to calm myself down, guzzling the air, reminding myself of the way Jarrod hung on my every word. I was different now, I told myself. I was powerful and lovable and worthy. Wasn't I?

"Hello?"

But when I heard his voice, that same voice that used to laugh at me for not being a real woman, the voice that used to terrorize me with stories of his more fulfilling escapades, I transformed into a pool of emotional goo.

When he didn't recognize my voice, I did my best to remind him who I was, mentioning where we met, where I lived, and what I looked like, as if a decade had passed instead of a year. Then I asked if he wanted to catch up. He sighed long and torturously before agreeing, "OK, sure."

Then he said, "My girlfriend is working late on Thursday. I can see you then." The word *girlfriend* coming out of his mouth made the idea urgent. I needed to make him mine. I agreed to meet him at 9:00 p.m., at some park I'd never heard of in Granada Hills, about an hour's drive from my house.

I considered my last sex session with Jarrod to be more for his benefit than mine—a gift. But when I watched him break down in tears, I realized who was really benefiting. I just couldn't figure out why. It didn't matter. On Thursday, I knew it would all be worthwhile. I'd finally fuck Alex, he'd break up with his girlfriend, and we'd live happily ever after.

On Thursday, I drove the hour to Granada Hills and made my way to the poorly lit park, listening to some of my favorite sappy love songs from the early 2000s. Lifehouse, Dido, and Coldplay, back-to-back-to-back.

I couldn't keep from trembling as I waited in my car. I felt sick. I'd popped only one of the pills Jarrod had given me because I wanted to feel relaxed but not completely numb. I needed to be fully aware of everything happening with Alex, so I could successfully turn it all around.

He showed up about a half hour late, pulling his car next to mine in the darkness. Filled with excitement tangled up with dread, I jumped out of my car and ran over to his.

He was smiling, which comforted me. He was glad to see me, I thought. This isn't a mistake. And when he got out of the car and pulled my body close to his, I thought I might collapse there. It was warm and perfect and I wanted desperately for it to be mine.

"It's been awhile," he said.

"Too long," I murmured.

But that's when I saw, just over his shoulder in the backseat of his car, a child's car seat and scattered toys.

"What's that?" I asked, pulling away from his body.

"What?" He glanced behind him.

"Do you have a kid?" I asked.

He laughed, turning back to face me. "Oh, you don't care that I have a girlfriend, but you care if I have a kid?"

"Yes, I care," I said. "I care that you have a girlfriend, and I care that you have a kid."

He narrowed his eyes as if I couldn't be serious. Then he reached into his car and got a bottle of wine before slamming the door shut. "I don't have a kid," he said, handing me the bottle. "Let's go for a walk in the park. C'mon."

I looked at the seat and then back at him. "You're not lying, right?"

Then he grabbed my face and pulled me close again, kissing me so intensely I thought I might fall over.

"Let's go," he said.

I followed him to the grass, which was wet when we sat down, and we took swigs from the bottle. There was so much I wanted to say to him, to show him how smart I was now, how much more womanly I'd become, but I held my voice inside myself and it seemed to die in there. It wasn't long before we were lying down on the grass and he was on top of me. He pulled down my jeans and started jabbing me with his fingers. That hurt, but I didn't say so. I just shifted my body around and moaned.

"This is what you wanted, right? This is why you drove down here?" He breathed hard into my neck.

I wanted him badly, but I couldn't stop thinking about that child's seat in the back of his car or imagining what his child might look like. Was it a boy or a girl? Did he or she have his blue eyes? What was his girlfriend like? I thought about Jarrod, too, the memory of him on his bed, and me, this wicked person I was becoming.

When his pants were down to his ankles, I started inching away, my bare ass slipping against the grass. "Hold on, wait," I said.

He kept kissing me, though, trying to pin me down with his hips. "C'mon, don't do this to me. You've come all this way."

"Just tell me you don't have a kid," I said. "Tell me you don't love your girlfriend. I need to hear it."

He pulled away, annoyed. "Why?"

"Because I don't want to just have sex with you and never see you again. I want this to be real."

"Oh God." He pulled his pants up and sat next to me on the grass. I sat up too. "What does it matter? You want to be my *girlfriend*?" The way he said *girlfriend* was in a baby voice, mocking me.

"I don't sound like that," I said softly, fastening the button on my jeans.

He shook his head. "I don't even know if you're a good fuck." Then he put the bottle back to his lips and finished it off.

"You don't have to talk to me that way," I said, trying to articulate an ounce of self-respect, but I was already too far in. I hated myself and he could see it.

"Look, I don't have time for this." He tossed the bottle away so that it rolled down a slope and we couldn't see it anymore.

"I'm not a virgin anymore," I assured him, as if it mattered.

"Congratulations?" He got up and started walking back to the car.

"Wait," I said. "I love you." I was disgusted with myself.

He gave me a look of pity and shook his head, lowering himself into his car and driving away from me, back to his life.

I wish I could say this was the last time I saw men like him, men dug up from a painful corner of my past and messily transposed onto a promising present to confirm the story I was intent on telling myself: this is all I deserve.

The next day, I found myself lost in my own neighborhood, driving around in circles and afraid to go home. I'd taken more pills than usual, but I wasn't sure how many. Not wanting to upset my parents, I called Jarrod and told him I needed his help. He told me to go to his house and he'd fix it.

By the time I made it there, I was hysterical. I told him the pills were making me crazy and I'd taken too many. I never knew what the pills were, but he didn't seem to know either.

"I think most of them are for anxiety and depression," he said. And then he added, "Some of them might be for pain."

"So you don't even know?" I yelled back.

"No, I'm sorry," he said, looking genuinely worried. "But you kept asking me for them and I gave you what I could find. I just wanted to make you happy." He started to cry.

I couldn't argue with that. I knew I'd been pushy about the pills. I'd been pushy about everything. I collapsed on his bed and sobbed.

"I'm an awful person," I told him. I wanted to confess about the night before, about the fool I'd made of myself, but I knew it would only upset him, and I couldn't upset him now. I needed him to take care of me.

He rubbed the back of my head while I cried into his pillow. "I love you," he said. "I don't think you're an awful person."

But his words only hurt me more, because I knew they weren't what I wanted. What I wanted didn't want me back. I got up from the bed, ran to my purse, and took the rest of the pills, eight or nine more, before he could stop me. He was screaming now, asking me why I'd done what I'd done, asking if we should go to the hospital.

We didn't go to the hospital. Instead, he fetched a bucket and I vomited up the pills before having dazed sex with him. Afterward, he dropped me off at home in my car and walked back to his house.

The next morning, I fainted in the shower before vomiting more, and then I called my mom to tell her what had happened. She rushed home in tears, demanding to know everything. Where had I gotten the pills? Why would I do such a thing?

But I couldn't explain. Everything sounded so melodramatic. This guy I liked didn't like me back. I didn't like this other guy who liked me. All I could do was tell her that I was trying to get high and that Jarrod was to blame.

"He's no longer welcome in this house," she decided, wiping her tears away. "Make sure he knows that."

◆

Though I felt ashamed of how things had ended with Jarrod and for letting my mom think he was to blame for all my toxic actions, I didn't offer an apology or try to remain friends. Instead, I ignored his phone calls and pretended I wasn't home whenever he dropped by my house.

When summer arrived, I reconnected with one of my high school friends, Laura, and turned all my attention to her. She, too, was enrolled at the same college, and I found her less intimidating than most other girls because I didn't feel the pressure to reveal too much of myself to her. Petite but feisty and full of energy, Laura was opinionated about everything and filled our time with endless chatter.

She knew various doormen at some of the hippest bars in Hollywood, and I'd drive us there in my Mustang with the top down, blasting "Magic Man" by Heart and all the No Doubt albums. At the cool bars in Hollywood, we'd exchange hugs and kisses with the doormen for the privilege of drinking without valid ID. I'd order a screwdriver and she'd order a peach schnapps, and when we were buzzed enough, we'd smile at older guys across the bar, smoke cigarettes with them out on the sidewalk, and sometimes exchange phone numbers. After we'd had enough, I'd drive us home, careful to keep my car within the lanes to make it there without getting a DUI. I considered her my best friend and convinced myself that intimacy was easy; I just needed the social lubricant that was so readily available in a $10 glass tumbler.

Together we decided to sign up for a study abroad trip to Italy in the fall. We'd seen the posters all around campus and I couldn't think of a better way to reinvent myself than world travel.

"I'm not sure," my mom said when I first told her about the trip. "Will you be safe out there?"

I rolled my eyes, feeling like a child begging to play outside, although I understood her concern. Her daughter had become a pill popper right under her roof and she hadn't even noticed. What else would she miss with me so far away?

"I promise everything will be OK," I assured her. "It'll be good for me."

◆

More than six thousand miles away from everything I knew and had grown bored with, what I remember most about Florence, besides the way the light hit the Ponte Vecchio at sunset and the endless green shutters that lined the streets, is my boyfriend Matt holding his finger over the shot hole of a hash pipe, telling me not to exhale.

Matt and I hooked up my first night in Florence, when Laura and I invited some of the guys from our group back to our apartment to drink. He had a lip ring and burgundy hair and played the guitar. He looked like Renton, Ewan McGregor's character in the movie *Trainspotting*, and this was no accident. It was his favorite film. I remember how he wasn't wearing a belt that first night and how I couldn't stop staring at his blue boxers covered in white stars.

While drinking would become a main component of my time in Italy, making me feel social and normal with my classmates in nightclubs and at parties and other terrifyingly shared spaces, getting stoned and fucking Matt took precedence.

We smoked hash he bought from gypsies at Santo Spirito, and pot we later picked up from coffee shops we traveled to in Amsterdam, smuggling it back to Florence in peanut butter jars. We got high all the time. Why study our Italian conjugations when we could get baked and sit for hours in the Piazza della Signoria, watching the city walk by? Why see the *David* in the Accademia Gallery when we could hit the bong again and order a pizza? We were so stoned that when they televised the 9/11 attacks on the news that somber afternoon, we thought the whole thing was fake.

Pot still made me feel uneasy and painfully analytical when I was around people, and so I preferred drinking when I was being social, but I loved smoking pot before sex with Matt. I had happily discovered that being high made my orgasms longer and more intense.

When I was stoned, my climax seemed almost everlasting, peak toppled upon peak, my brain and body flooded with undistracted pleasure. Physical sensations were heightened so that I had no interest in my racing thoughts as soon as my clothes were off and Matt was touching me. Orgasms felt new, nearly as significant as those very first ones in that bathtub at twelve. One time, I even cried. It was embarrassing, even though Matt didn't tease me about it. He just made me come again.

Matt, a twenty-year-old white boy from an affluent neighborhood in LA, who had cigarette burns on his arms he'd inflicted on himself and homemade tattoos, became a symbol of everything I deemed edgy and rebellious and desirable. He talked about his friends back home who played in bands and had drug habits and sometimes got into trouble with the law. And, I thought to myself, *How exciting, how dangerous*, and felt cool by association. Besides serving as a gateway into pot smoking on a regular basis, because Matt wanted to have sex as often as I did, *he* also became my new drug.

Even though I lived with Laura, our friendship was no longer as important to me, and she didn't seem to mind. My interest also waned in touring the endless museums and historic sites Florence offered. Sure, I saw Elizabeth Barrett Browning's bed and Dante's old house. I watched an authentic Italian opera and climbed the steps to the top of Il Duomo. We took long train rides to Oktoberfest in Munich and snapped photos at the top of the Eiffel Tower. But none of these things would've been even slightly appealing had Matt not been there right beside me. While Laura and other classmates were bonding over gelatos in city squares and day trips to the exotic islands of Italy, I was slipping into severe codependency.

I wanted nothing but to show Matt that I cared. When the three-month trip was over and we returned to LA, we both decided to major in English and take all our classes together at our community college. And whenever we weren't in class, we behaved just as we had in Italy—smoking weed all through the afternoon and having sex. I was happy for the most part, and completely enamored of him, but I couldn't shake a new fear from slithering around in my brain: *When is this going to end? When is he going to leave me?*

If I caught him smiling at the waitress when he ordered food or looking into the checkout girl's eyes at the grocery store, I'd think to myself that he wanted to fuck her. Then I'd imagine their bodies doing all the things *our* bodies did now and I'd feel sick with jealousy.

I also felt threatened by his past, which seemed far superior to mine because he was white. He kept photos of his pretty ex-girlfriends up in his room next to photos of him and his pack of friends, most of them looking high and happy and fun and normal. He'd tried drugs I'd always been too scared to try—ecstasy, acid, and mushrooms. His stories from the past, which used to excite me, now threatened me. He was experimental. I was not. He was cool. I was a poser. And although he'd only slept with one more person than I had, I couldn't help from feeling like he had a sexual advantage over me, that maybe I wasn't as good as I thought he was in bed. As much as I tried to stow away this feeling of inadequacy in the back of my mind, it always came back with a vengeance. I obsessed about when he would cheat on me, what it would feel like to lose him, and how damaged I would be as a result.

My remedy to this was to wow him with my sexual prowess, to prove to him I was an adventurous, insatiable vixen always down to fuck. Then how could he leave me? All his friends would give him shit if he did. *Didn't she want to suck your dick all the time? You fucked up, bro!* I had to prove I was better than his ex-girlfriends, whom I thought were prettier than me, and any other girl I saw him talking to or looking at.

So I returned to the source of it all: porn.

Porn would teach me how to deep throat without gagging, how to squeeze my tits together when he was on top to keep them from sliding into my armpits, how to talk dirty, and how much hotter it was to swallow his cum instead of spitting it out.

We were stoned, as usual, when I first suggested Matt and I watch porn together.

"Are you sure?" he asked. He looked confused.

"Yeah, I love porn. Here, let me show you some of my favorites."

I went to his computer, opened one of my go-to sites and typed in a few random search terms to lead us to some clips I thought he might like. I chose one of a secretary with big tits sucking her boss's dick under his desk to get a raise. From then on, we had a new component to our pot and sex sessions. And when we weren't watching porn clips, we were making our own with his digital camera. Sometimes, we'd have sex while watching ourselves have sex, and I'd study my movements with an eagle's eye, thinking, *Next time, I'll suck in my tummy when I'm on top. I better shave those stray hairs I missed on my thighs.*

Years later, I'd shudder to think of the whereabouts of these videos and others like them I'd film over time. And all those photos too. My body, at different stages of life, captured by handheld camcorder or cell phone. Sent, with naive trust and compliance, over email and text message. And saved, for however long the recipient wanted, on computer hard drive, USB stick, photo album, and memory. When the term *revenge porn* started popping up everywhere and websites on "slutty exgirlfriends" became common, I developed a new kind of fear and regret. Would the day come where I'd click from one link to the next and find a harrowing image of some past version of myself?

Although we were having a lot of sex, and I found this sex fulfilling, I somehow found myself always wanting more from Matt when it was over. It quickly became clear to me that I wasn't just playing the role of an insatiable vixen to make him stay. I *was* insatiable. After he'd fall into a post-orgasm slumber, I'd give myself a few more orgasms until I was exhausted. Only then could I fall asleep beside him.

When we were separated—he still lived with his parents, and I still lived with mine—I obsessed about when I would see him again, calling him every few hours, needing to know his whereabouts at all times. If he didn't answer, I drove myself mad with worry. *Who is he with? What is he doing? Why isn't he spending time with me?*

One day, more than a year into dating, I found a printout of driving directions in his car. At first, he said he didn't remember what they were for, but after pushing him, he confessed that he went to a party with his friend Sam a few weeks before. I was furious, imagining him getting stoned or drunk and flirting with girls, pretending he was single without me.

"Did you fuck anyone?" I screamed at him.

"What? Of course not! I just hung out with Sam."

"But you lied to me!" I yelled back.

"I lied because I knew you'd be pissed. I just wanted to hang out with my friends for the night."

This idea enraged me. That he would choose his friends over me. That he would lie to me in order to do so. What else was he lying about? Who else would he choose over me?

I had him drive me home and I told him I needed space. When I was inside my house, I tried to distract myself from my thumping heart and racing thoughts by masturbating, and this was effective for a few minutes, until I came, and then I got angry all over again. I did this a few more times, watching porn to help me along, but every time I came and returned to myself, I returned to the fury. I wasn't cooling down. So I dialed Matt up and yelled at him some more, telling him he was a liar, an asshole, a cheater, a pothead, a loser, and everything else I could think up in my anger.

Annoyed, he hung up on me, but I just dialed again. He hung up. I dialed again. I was in the middle of another rant and he was calling me crazy, when my mom opened my bedroom door.

"I'm on the phone," I told her, holding my cell phone against my chest. But she looked distraught. I could tell she'd been crying.

"Hang up," she said.

"I have to go," I told Matt, hanging up before he could say anything else. "What's up?"

She stood there for a second, silently. I held my breath.

"Jarrod."

That's what she said. Not "something happened to Jarrod," or "there's been an accident," or anything else true and telling. Just his name, hanging there between us like a chandelier, delicate and beautiful, but a bit too much.

"What about him?" I asked, sitting down slowly on the bed, scared to move too fast, scared to hear what could only make her look this way.

She just shook her head. "He's dead."

"What?" I started to laugh in panic. "No, c'mon, that's not true." I stood up again and immediately dialed his number. "I just saw him the other day."

This was mostly true. Jarrod had dropped by my house about a month before, only I didn't talk to him. I was in my room, talking on the phone with Matt, when my mom knocked on my door to tell me Jarrod was out front and wanted to show me his new motorcycle. Now that I had a new boyfriend and Jarrod was no longer a threat, she was friendly to him, but I didn't want to be friendly to him. I told her to tell him I wasn't home.

"But your car is out front," she whispered, so he wouldn't hear us talking about him from the front door.

I just shrugged. I didn't care. Then I peeked through my curtains and watched him go back to his motorcycle and speed away, not knowing that would be the last time I'd ever see him.

His grandma answered the phone after a few rings, but when I asked to speak to him, her response confirmed the news. "I'm sorry, but Jarrod was in a motorcycle accident. He passed away."

I hung up without saying good-bye. What does a person say after that? *I'm sorry*? The words were far too little and far too late. But I was sorry. I was horribly sorry. I was more sorry than I had ever been about anything before.

◆

About a month after Jarrod's death, my mom came into my room to find me facedown in a tangle of sheets. She'd been making an almost hourly inquiry into my mental health since the tragedy, as I didn't seem to be coping. I'd stopped eating, stopped going to classes, and I'd lash out at her, my dad, and Matt when they tried to help. I'd only let my sister, Ashley, crawl into bed with me sometimes, although at ten, she couldn't truly understand what was going on. My grief stretched far beyond missing Jarrod or feeling sad about his unfortunate fate. I was consumed with unrelenting guilt and shame. I couldn't stop the flashbacks from crashing into my mind. The things I said to him, the way I'd laughed at him, the carelessness with which I'd treated his love. I wanted nothing but to go back and tell him I was sorry.

Seeing me there, hopeless, my mom put her warm hand on my back. "I know you're going through a lot," she said, "but there's someone I want you to see."

I didn't want to see anyone, but I needed a solution. "Who?"

"She's a healer. And she . . ." She hesitated.

"She what?"

"You're going to think it sounds crazy," she said, looking away from me as I turned my face up to her. "She can speak to the dead."

I quickly sat up in bed. "When can I see her?"

Montebello was not the sort of place that embraced healers or clairvoyants. When Joy opened her wellness center amid the city's strip malls and taquerias, it was an anomaly. She brought yoga, Reiki, hypnosis, past-life regression, and other spiritual practices to a city that couldn't have been less ready for it. Thus, her business only lasted a few months, but in those few months I was her enthusiastic disciple.

Joy had a warm presence about her that was free of judgment. She made me feel safe, like even if I confided a violent crime to her with gruesome details, she'd still find me deserving of compassion and love. In her center, surrounded by Buddha statues, paintings of Ganesha, and the aroma of incense, I found a calmness that I hadn't felt since those times I tried to meditate back in high school. She introduced me to yoga, which felt like a mini vacation from the misery. She taught me positive affirmations. And as far as reaching Jarrod, she offered only simple reassurances. That all was forgiven. That no resentment lived inside him and it never had. That I should be gentle on myself. And merciful. It wasn't much, but it was exactly what I needed to hear.

When Joy's place closed down and she moved to Arizona, where the economic prospects were better, I closed down that part of myself that had started to open up to grace.

That fall I was accepted as a transfer student to UCLA, despite my slipping grades. Matt was accepted too. We decided to move closer to campus, he to university housing in Westwood and me to a loft apartment in Culver City.

What I didn't realize was that my time with Joy had resulted in a shift that could not be undone no matter how hard I would try to evade it. Even though I would return to my destructive patterns, and develop worse ones in time, a seed had been planted. The question was: When would I care enough to help it grow?

six

THE FLEEING GIRL

Moving over to the west side in the summer of 2003, Matt threw himself into the college social scene, bonding with the other students in his university housing, which was noisy and smoke-filled and as intimidating as I'd always imagined dorms to be. I spent most of my time envying his ability to make new friends. Now that I lived away from my parents, I didn't have to go to Matt's house for pot and sex. I bought myself a bong and a vibrator and edged away from him, preferring my own apartment to nurse my habits of escapism.

Located so close to Interstate 10 that the whole place rattled when trucks drove past, my apartment had a loft, where I hid out, and a bedroom downstairs occupied by an aspiring actress with Kenyan roots. I hated the feeling of sharing my personal space with another woman, especially a woman like her—tall, big-breasted, confident, and talented. Luckily Jade was often at casting calls or with her boyfriend, so our interactions were limited to brief encounters in the kitchen where she'd ask me repeatedly to stop smoking in the house. I'd smile politely, apologize, and then climb the stairs to my loft to piss her off again. Nobody was going to tell me what I could or could not do in my place, and anyway, I didn't plan on staying there forever.

When I wasn't in my little nest, I was on campus, studying my ass off. From Chaucer to Shakespeare to Austen, I read everything required that would earn me a bachelor's degree in English at UCLA with honors, and I was on an academic plan to finish in one year, after which I'd decided I would return to Europe without Matt. I imagined Europe would be the place I would not only be a serious reader—since that's what I thought college had made of me—but also a serious writer. I wanted literary greatness; I just didn't think I had lived enough to write about anything worthwhile.

I also got a part-time job as a bookseller at Barnes & Noble, where I mainly worked the children's section, answering the question "Do you have *Goodnight Moon*?" multiple times a day and neatly reshelving board books every time they were once again scattered across the aisles. While Matt was making friends with fellow classmates, I was making my own friends at the bookstore. This quickly became a point of contention because I only made friends with men.

In an attempt to make Matt jealous and convince myself that I could get over my social awkwardness if I tried, I often invited these men back to my apartment to drink. Sometimes these nights would end up with me lounging on my bed until I was too drunk to make a coherent sentence. Having been paranoid for so long about Matt cheating on me, I was adamant about fidelity, even when I playfully touched knees and hugged a little longer than I should've and talked openly about my favorite sexual positions. When they were gone, I'd masturbate until I was exhausted, fantasizing about each of them taking turns on me like I'd seen in various gang-bang clips.

Sometimes I hung out with Laura, but we had little to talk about unless we were drinking, smoking weed, or gossiping about people from high school we didn't know anymore. If ever I felt myself opening up to her about Jarrod, Matt, my future, or anything else that caused my breath to shorten, my chest to tighten, or my heart to beat harder than normal, she'd change the subject to something lighter. I quickly learned that it wasn't cool to share that much. I shouldn't be a downer.

She wasn't the only one who thought I was a downer. Matt often complained about my pessimism, encouraging me to see the bright side of things if he noticed my thoughts taking a dark turn. He'd pack up the pipe and take off his pants, and only then could I shut off my brain.

"Maybe you should find another hippie lady like that one near your house," he said one day, when I wouldn't stop complaining about how bored I felt in LA. Then he laughed at the idea, because things like yoga and meditation went way over his head. He didn't know what else to offer me though. I was chronically dissatisfied and sure he was growing tired of me.

When I announced I was leaving for London after my graduation, knowing he still had another year to go, his response wasn't relief like I'd expected.

"Just wait another year," he pleaded. "I can finish up and join you. It'll be just like Florence."

But I didn't want things to be like Florence. I wanted a fresh start, which entailed leaving it all behind—Matt, LA, and all the memories stored there—even if it meant hurting him to do so. I convinced myself it was better this way, like ripping off a Band-

Aid. It was only a matter of time before I fucked it up, I thought. It was only a matter of time before I hurt him the way I hurt Jarrod or he hurt me. Both were frightening prospects. It was safer to walk away.

◆

I signed up for a monthlong course to teach English as a foreign language at a London language school in the fall of 2004, giving my parents the peace of mind that I wouldn't be squandering their money. I was making an exciting career choice, I told them. And so I set off for the city of Virginia Woolf and George Orwell, though I felt more like Sylvia Plath or T. S. Eliot, an expat whose real mission was to escape. The idea of practice teaching—standing before a group of people as an authority figure—was terrifying and not entirely what I wanted, but I was up for the challenge if it meant changing my city, my relationship status, and, ultimately, my life.

Before the course began, I stayed in a hotel my first week in London, relishing long walks through the quirky backstreets of Notting Hill and along the Thames, and drinking tea alone in cafés while I wrote. There was peace in spending time with my thoughts and exploring unfamiliar streets, and with no plans or people to constrict me, I indulged in the freedom of doing only what pleased me, whether it was heading to the National Gallery or staying in bed late to read. Having fallen for "The Love Song of J. Alfred Prufrock" and "The Waste Land" in college, I carried only one book around with me—*The Collected Poems of T.S. Eliot 1909–1935*—and I read these poems over and over, finding new intricacies to love each time. The hotel didn't have internet access, and I hadn't saved any porn on my laptop, but I surprised myself when I didn't miss the slutty secretaries, the naughty nurses, or the cock-hungry cheerleaders. It also didn't matter that I didn't know anyone; I slipped into anonymity with pleasure.

Walking through the streets of London, peering into unfamiliar shops, and imagining myself as a real writer instilled in my head a new version of myself that I liked. And every time I planted myself in new cities and situations across the globe thereafter, I'd be reminded of this alter ego, which was enough to empower me to overcome my habits and do something, anything, besides what I was used to. What I didn't understand then was the temptation of relapse looming nearby. Caught up in the sunny patches of new beginnings, it was difficult to see how easily it could all crumble again.

During the first week of the course, I realized just how challenging this venture would be. Not only was the workload heavy—we were expected to be there five days a week, from 9:00 a.m. to 6:00 p.m., creating lesson plans, writing up reports, and taking turns teaching various levels of English—the course was also heavy on collaboration. As usual, I found discomfort in the group—obsessed with being perceived as cool, interesting, smart, and pretty—but after a few lunches and brainstorms, I calmed down and actually enjoyed spending time with my classmates. They seemed to enjoy spending time with me too. New possibilities entered my mind—could I be comfortable in social situations? Could I be worthy of friendship and fun?

Liam was a gay guy from Ireland who bonded with me over Morrissey. Sandra, a painter, would join me for sushi lunches, where we'd talk about art and our ex-boyfriends. Will always had a new joke to tell, only Haley's jokes were dirtier. But it was Anna who I loved spending most of my time with. She was beautiful, funny, and affectionate, and after hearing how much money my parents were spending on my hotel, she offered an extra room at her parents' house, where she was living.

"I can introduce you to all my friends," she said. "And my parents will love you!"

I happily agreed.

Anna's home was in Blackheath Village, a suburb in Southeast London near Greenwich. The place had an old piano and scores of interesting books, and always smelled like freshly baked bread. Anna's parents, Elizabeth and Richard, despite being church people, were loose, lively, and well educated. This surprised me because I had convinced myself long ago that only ignorant people believed in God. Christianity was for sheep. But they weren't sheep. Elizabeth was a well-read psychologist, and Richard had lived all over the world before settling in London. He was full of adventurous stories and his face lit up when he told them.

Anna, along with her three sisters who didn't live at home anymore, was raised to live a life of charity and faith. This meant that she held Bible-study meetings in her living room and sang in the church choir several times a week. Sometimes when I made myself dinner in the kitchen, I heard her and the girls in her Bible study laughing together from the other room, a sense of warm camaraderie filling the house. She often invited me to join them, but I always politely declined, having no interest in returning to my oppressive Catholic roots.

Sometimes she'd practice church songs on the piano, calling me in to sit beside her and sing along. When she first asked, I remember feeling far too shy and self-conscious, even though I remembered the songs from childhood. Only when she insisted and promised to sing with me, saying it would help her practice, did I agree. To my surprise, I enjoyed singing, the sound of my voice holding steady and strong with hers. The songs also tapped into memories I thought I'd long forgotten, back to when God seemed less like a tyrant in the sky and more like a reliable source of love and forgiveness. Though it was hard to rationalize in my intellectual mind, which had grown wary of organized religion, I came to look forward to the times Anna asked me to join her at the piano, or to accompany her to Sunday mass with her parents, after which she'd link arms with me and we'd walk home, laughing together and sharing stories. I couldn't tell what I appreciated more—being connected to something sacred, or to her.

Anna was also the first girl I'd ever met who was in her twenties and still a virgin. Although she'd ask me questions about my past relationships and listen with unfeigned interest, she seemed completely confident, and even happy, with her decision to save herself for marriage.

"But don't you wonder what it's like?" I once asked, genuinely confused how someone could wait so long.

She just shrugged. "Of course, but it can wait. I don't feel deprived."

I remember how my face got hot when she said this because I couldn't forget how deprived I'd felt before sex and how deprived I still felt. I thought back to the sex, the porn, and the sexual fantasies that had, for so long, dominated my mind and I wondered if she could tell what was going on with me. Did she think I was a bad person? Did she feel sorry for me?

She grabbed my hand.

"I don't judge you, if that's what you're thinking," she said. "Everybody's on a different path, and I think you're incredible."

In an instant, I felt better. I felt accepted.

Just because Anna had never had sex and just because she was devoted to her faith, this doesn't mean she wasn't any fun. We shared bottles of wine while blasting the *Moulin Rouge* soundtrack, dancing in her living room through the night. She also took me to various parties and bars with her group of friends, and I felt surprisingly confident in these spaces. I even toted around my book of Eliot's poems and I read lines when I felt inspired. Nobody seemed to mind my literary geekiness. I felt friendly and interesting, and this encouraged me to share more of myself, making conversation something to be excited about, instead of something to be feared.

The thought of watching porn sometimes crept into my mind, but I simply didn't have access anymore. There was no Wi-Fi in Anna's house, which meant that if I wanted to watch it, I would have to do so on the living room computer, and I didn't want to risk getting caught. Instead, I masturbated under the covers when I was alone at night, but even this was rare. I often found myself too exhausted from coursework to act out.

When the course ended, I found myself with a lot of extra time, and fearing that I might overstay my welcome at Anna's house, I rented another room in the next neighborhood over. The new place had three other roommates, and while they were all kind, I didn't find them approachable. When they weren't working, they spent most of their time alone in their rooms, making the shared spaces quiet and cold, and the living situation isolating. I found the move jarring. Without Anna's warm and positive energy holding me up throughout the day, I felt lonely and less confident in myself.

I still saw Anna, but less frequently, and she was leaving soon anyway to teach in India. The idea of being on my own in London again, as thrilling as it had been upon arrival, now felt scary. I had grown accustomed to this happy and confident persona of mine, but I wouldn't take credit for it. *I only became this person because of Anna,* I thought. She was a good influence on me and now she was leaving. The only way to hang on to her and the person I had become was to cling to people she knew. Now, when we met up at bars, I chose to sit by her male friends, seeing them as more reliable prospects for consistent affection and attention.

I started sleeping with Paul, a history teacher who cooked me dinners from a Jamie Oliver cookbook. He told me I gave the best head he'd ever had. And when he wasn't available, I hung out with Daniel, who bought me drinks, took me ice-skating, and sometimes went down on me. Not sleeping with him or returning oral sex were deliberate decisions I made so that I didn't seem like a slut, especially since they were both Anna's friends.

But I didn't stop at Anna's friends. I also started spending time with a photographer named Craig, who was a friend of one of my new roommates. After showing me some of his London landscape photographs one evening, he asked if I would pose for some portraits and I agreed.

In his studio, after hours, he suggested I pose without my clothes, giving me baby oil to rub all over my body. I remember his erection showing through his pants while he snapped photos, and the pit in my stomach that grew as I removed one article of clothing after the next. I felt as if each article I removed was like taking one step further away from that girl in the bar reading T. S. Eliot poems and walking arm in arm with Anna. Spreading my legs for the camera, it felt familiar and depressing to return to an old idea: *This is how you get people to like you.*

◆

After Christmas rolled around, my parents broke the news that they wouldn't be financially supporting me anymore. They said I should think about putting my teaching English as a foreign language (TEFL) certification to use like I said I would. I knew then that it was only a matter of time before my London adventure would be over. I couldn't legally work abroad and, anyway, I'd never had any intention of using my TEFL certification. I had no choice but to return to LA.

If I thought moving just blocks away from Anna's house was jarring, nothing could have prepared me for what I felt moving back home. It was like coming down from a high, the high of independence, and suddenly I had no idea what to do with myself. Every time my mom asked me to do the dishes, I felt like I was twelve years old again. I got a job as an English tutor but only worked about five hours a week, so I made very little money. When I didn't work, I tried to write about London, but searching my memories only made me miss the city and I'd end up feeling angry with myself for leaving.

Being back in Montebello also roused all sorts of unresolved feelings about Jarrod. I felt as if his death had occurred days before, instead of two years. Just as my brain slipped back into its old habit of feeling guilty and ashamed, my body slipped back into its old habits as well. I turned to porn, masturbation, drinking, and a new venture—casual sex.

With the help of Myspace, people from the past were now conveniently present whenever I searched their names. Guys I'd met with Laura at those cool bars in Hollywood. Fellow classmates I'd been friendly to in college. I had sex with Adam after a concert at the Hollywood Palladium. I slept with Keith in San Francisco when I was supposed to be bonding with my brother. I hooked up with a waiter/actor named Peter for months, and over the course of those months, we made several trips to Planned Parenthood, to pick up Plan B or take pregnancy tests. Fucking without condoms gave sex an extra charge, and we were both hopelessly hooked on it.

But I spent most of my time with Ben and Simon, who were brothers. They lived in Pico Rivera, just five minutes away from my parents' house, played in a band, and loved to drink. I'd invite them over and they'd bring along jugs of cheap tequila and, sometimes, girls they were dating, girls they'd get me to make out with when the tequila made us brave enough. My parents had always loved throwing parties, and they were famous for drinking all night without suffering hangovers in the morning, so they didn't mind when we filled the house with drunken laughter, blasting music and splashing around in the pool, before passing out in random spots around the house. We'd do this two, three, sometimes four times a week.

During those nights, I was talkative and funny and I liked this version of myself. I felt normal. After I'd had enough tequila and was feeling ballsy, I'd rave about the kind of porn I liked, but I'd refrain from mentioning clips I thought they'd consider too gross.

My preferences were changing all the time. I loved "old and young" clips. I'd also taken a liking to watching drunken girls get walked around on leashes at parties or get fucked by groups of men while seemingly unconscious. I'd discovered the category "bukkake" and felt simultaneously disgusted and excited every time I watched multiple men come all over a girl's face before urging her to lick up the drips that had fallen on the carpet beneath her. I didn't consider any of this normal, so I talked about threesomes and strippers instead. Schoolgirls and slutty milfs and other categories I didn't find stimulating anymore.[12]

---

12 Gary Wilson, author of *Your Brain on Porn: Internet Pornography and the Emerging Science of Addiction*, who is probably most famous for his TEDxGlasgow talk, "The Great Porn Experiment," has found that watching too much porn in adolescence has trained the brain to need everything associated with porn to get aroused. And because online porn clips are endless and easily accessible, users can click from scene to scene, corresponding with the ebbs and flows of their arousal, training the brain to depend heavily on novelty.

Sometimes I took out my laptop and played some of the "nicer" clips as if I were simply turning on the radio. And every time I did these things, or confessed to hating condoms, or to having an un- usually high sex drive, I hoped the guys liked me even more than they seemed to. I was one of them, I thought, and not like other girls. When my confessions would elicit laughs or high fives or nods of recognition, I'd feel a rush of what I thought was intimacy.

My sister, Ashley, would sometimes join in on the fun when my parents were asleep or out of the house, even though she was just thirteen at the time. I'd sneak her shots of tequila and the guys would laugh, telling me what a bad sister I was. But I thought the opposite. Knowing what it felt like to be left out by my brother, Gabe, and all my male cousins when I was younger, I didn't want her to go through that. I told myself I was doing her a favor, and I imagined her thanking me in the future. I aimed to be the coolest big sister anyone ever had.

During one of these drunken pool parties, I hooked up with one of the brothers, Simon. When we woke up together the next day, I was consumed with regret. I wanted the brothers to think of me as one of them, not as one of their interchangeable girl- friends. The girlfriends, I imagined, lived in some polarized and inferior place outside of us. But sleeping with Simon, against my best wishes, quickly became a usual thing. So did the cringing that came every time I woke up sober and naked beside him. When he started coming around without his brother, I tried to make it clear that I wasn't interested in having a relationship and that it shouldn't happen again. Then we'd drink. It always happened again.

When he told me that he loved me, I told myself, *That's it, I'm stopping this.* Then we drank, fucked, and I ended up telling him I loved him too.

"This is going to ruin our friendship," I assured him one morning. "We need to stop."

"But what if it could become more than a friendship?" he pleaded. "You're not even giving us a chance."

"I don't want a relationship," I snapped. "I just want to have fun."

Then we started hooking up when we weren't drunk. His house, my house, motels, cars. I'd start dating a new guy, but when that got boring, I'd break things off and call up Simon. Then I'd go back to the guy I'd broken up with, and then back to Simon, like a Ping-Pong ball. This made him oscillate between sadness and fury. He left me voice mails cussing me out and emails full of accusations that I was a slut, I was damaged, I'd never be happy with anyone. These voice mails and emails were always followed by apologies and proclamations of his love.

"I love you," he said in one of his voice mails. "But you're driving me crazy. Either be with me or let me get on with my life."

I couldn't understand why he wouldn't just accept our arrangement. I thought that's what men wanted. To have easy access to sex with no strings attached. He was making everything too complicated.

One night, I was out drinking alone, trying to minimize the time I spent with the brothers so I would stop sleeping with Simon. Across the bar, there was an unexpected sight—a group of my old teachers from high school. I could tell they had been drinking for some time already. They were loose and loud, no longer the stiff authority figures I remembered. They saw me, too, and invited me over to their table to drink.

At some point in the night, I must have blacked out, because I only remember fragments. Making out in a bar bathroom with a busty female teacher who'd given me high grades my sophomore year. Having her breast in my mouth when a customer walked in and told us to get a room. Drunkenly asking another one of my teachers, a man with a gray beard who was much older than me, what he'd do if he and I were alone in a hotel room together, and him saying: "I could think of a few things." Giving a blow job to a man whose face I can't visualize, in an apartment I don't recall driving to, while the same female teacher I'd made out with made me come with her tongue.

Whenever I was sober, flashbacks of my drunken activities haunted me throughout the day. I could never remember at what point of the night my sense rolled away from me, making bad decisions seem like good ones. But I was caught up in a cycle I didn't know how to escape.

The morning I decided to leave LA for Hawaii—where things would get completely out of control—I was suffering from a particularly troubling flashback from the previous night. My parents were out of town with Ashley, and the brothers were over with two male friends I'd never met. In my drunkenness, I couldn't figure out how to heat up the Jacuzzi out back, and so I told them to come to my parents' bathroom, where there was a jetted tub. I remember getting naked and splashing around in the bubbles while the guys stood there, drinks in hand, watching.

"Come in," I called to them, and they all did at some point, although we could barely fit. I remember grabbing at dicks under the water and Simon glaring at me. I remember drinking so much tequila I couldn't focus on whose mouth I was kissing from one moment to the next. And when I woke up naked the next day, alone and sickened with myself, I was too afraid to consider what I could not remember.

◆

My decision to go to Hawaii was inspired by surfer-turned-crooner Jack Johnson's album of love songs, *In Between Dreams*, which was huge in 2005 and the most uplifting album I'd ever owned. Jack was the antithesis of all the tragic music I usually listened to— devoted to the ocean and to the earth and, more important, to his wife of more than ten years. I wanted Jack's upbeat music to be the soundtrack to the next chapter of my life, which I hoped would be full of healthier choices. The move was equally inspired by a memory of myself I held tight to from a childhood vacation to Maui—a little girl in a flowery dress, my skin tanned, my feet in the sand, feeling happy and humble and in awe of the ocean.

I wanted to start over again, like I'd done in London, only this time I wouldn't ruin it. Hawaii, with its clean air and clear water and green mountains, would nurture me back to being a respectable person. I'd find that little girl again. After realizing I could run away without my parents' help by withdrawing all the money I'd ever saved as a waitress—about $6,000—I bought a one-way ticket and left. They were supportive of my decision to move, especially my mom.

"Make the most of it," she said. "One day you'll be married with kids and won't have this kind of freedom."

The first few days on the island, I stayed in an overpriced hotel room without air-conditioning in the touristy town of Lahaina. It was hot and cramped in there, so I knew I had to find a job quickly and get my own place. Luckily, it was easy to find work, so long as I wasn't picky.

After walking into a handful of restaurants with my beaming smile, I was hired as a cocktail waitress at a beachfront café. I spent a few hours a week serving mai tais, piña coladas, and other umbrella drinks to bikini-clad tourists and stoned surfers. It wasn't much money, but it was enough to rent a room.

I moved into a crowded house in Mahinahina, a neighborhood on the west side of Maui. The house was divided into separate apartments and rent was manageable—$700 a month. It was a shoe box of a room, only big enough for my bed and clothes, and the people who lived in the other apartments were like ghosts—I would hear them sometimes but rarely see them. Once in a while, I'd see Andrew, a real estate agent, cutting weeds in the front yard. Occasionally I'd see Tina, a hotel worker, wander from her room to the restroom or dillydally in the hallway. Bobby, a middle-aged guitarist, sometimes dropped by the kitchen before retreating to his place on the lanai.

It was Helen, the landlady, I saw most regularly. She was a petite, skinny Vietnamese woman in her late fifties who'd had a lot of work done. Facelift scars peeked through under her bob of shiny black hair, her tattooed eyebrows arched high on her wrinkle-free forehead, her breasts were perky, and she spoke with a thick accent.

I tried to be invisible in the house, being courteous but distant with my new roommates, and I tried to do the same at work. The restaurant was one nonstop party and the employees one big clique of friends who loved one another as much as they loved riding waves and getting drunk. The island was a magnet for free spirits and social butterflies. For the kind of people who displayed group photos on their fridge and always had a funny story to tell. It was the kind of place where everyone seemed comfortable wearing their bathing suits all day long, their athletic, tanned, and hairless bodies a daily reminder of what I only felt comfortable revealing after a few drinks, usually because it was the best thing I felt I had to offer.

Every day presented a new group outing and a new opportunity to make friends. A booze cruise, a beach bonfire, a volcano trek, a zip line adventure. And while I was invited to a few of these outings, I never went. I felt too awkward in the presence of their carefree laughter and happy faces. I tried to look happy too, but my smile felt forced. *I just need to adjust*, I told myself. *I'll be happy like them when I settle in.*

I craved feeling the way I'd felt those first weeks in London, open and friendly, but I feared that I was no longer that person. I still felt self-conscious and insecure, only now I had this voice in my head pressuring me to hurry up and be different. The voice was persistent and bullying, tearing me down if I smiled at someone or attempted small talk with my new coworkers, shouting, *Nobody likes you! You're a fake! You don't belong here!* I worried that whoever that girl was in London, that girl I'd caught a glimpse of, maybe she was an anomaly. Maybe I'd lost her.

The only relief from this voice in my head was my time away from the restaurant. I worked about three nights a week at four hours a shift. On my days off, I heard my landlady Helen's bedroom door open in the late morning or early afternoon when I was just waking. She'd make her way through her hanging door beads, head to the kitchen for a moment, and emerge with a piece of fruit or a slice of bread. She never cooked substantial meals for herself. Then she'd go back to her room to watch TV or drink wine or do both until it was time to go to the beach. Once in a while, she'd get dressed up and go out. I always knew when she was going out—the house smelled like perfume and a Sinatra album would be playing at full volume. Helen would sing along like an opera star, her accented howling filling the whole house. I'd go to the kitchen and see her through the door beads standing before the lit-up magnifying mirror, curling her eyelashes with one hand while a glass of red wine balanced in the other.

One night, she caught my glance and called me over. Her room had floor-to-ceiling windows that overlooked the ocean and it would've been the perfect view had a banana tree not blocked most of it.

"Why don't you go out?" she asked me as she swept the blush brush all over her face, along the scalp line, under the chin, everywhere. I'd been on the island for almost a month at this point but still hadn't made any friends.

"I'm writing all the time," I told her, which was true and usually my most acceptable excuse for not being social.

"What do you write about?"

"Oh," I hesitated, trying to think of something witty. I felt shy talking about the subjects of my writing. I didn't think I was a very good writer. At this time I mostly wrote as a way to remember things—how Elizabeth Barrett Browning's pillow had looked sunken in, like she'd just left her bed in her Florence apartment. Or as a way to remember feelings—how horrifying it had been to hear about Jarrod's death and how free I had felt to fly away from it all and land in London.

But I mostly wrote about the men in my life. Men I'd liked or kissed or fucked. Men I'd sat next to on trains or planes. Men I'd wanted to sit next to. I had a shitty memory when it came to phone numbers and names of songs and movies, but when it came to men, I had an almost photographic memory. Once a man entered my mind, it seemed he was lodged there forever. I liked to quiz myself on how much I could remember about each of them, filling my journals or Microsoft Word documents with scattered details of how they tasted in my mouth, the things they told me, how it felt to be held by them. I assigned significance to the most minute experiences so that I wouldn't forget, and I hoped in recording these experiences, they would somehow become more meaningful. That later, when I looked back, I would recall a life of passion and daring adventures instead of emptiness or embarrassment.

"I guess I write about everything. Life, traveling . . . men."

She blotted her lips with a tissue and turned to look at me. "You have a man?" When she said "man," her eyelids dropped a bit and she shot me a seductive gaze. I shook my head at her. Then she turned her back to me. "Get dressed. I'll treat you to dinner tonight." I hesitated, as I did with every invitation, then thought, *Screw it—it's free dinner.*

We went to a pricey French restaurant on the other side of the island, a little over a half-hour drive from Lahaina. We feasted on caviar, roasted duck, and pineapples filled with crème brûlée, courtesy of the owner, Luc, an older man who had once dated Helen in the eighties. Now they were just friends.

"I'm fickle," she told me, when I asked Helen if she'd ever been married. We were more than halfway through the bottle of champagne. "I have two grown daughters who live in Florida with very wealthy husbands." She paused and smiled. "They did good."

"Were you ever married to their father?" The more I drank the more I felt fine asking personal questions.

"Yes, I was married to him. And I was a good wife—stayed beautiful for him." She sipped her champagne slowly in between her confessions. "But I didn't love him. I don't love anyone. How about you?"

"How about me?"

"Do you love?"

But before I could answer, she cleared her throat. "Because you shouldn't," she said. "You're beautiful. You should have five boyfriends. One for each day of the week."

"How about the other two days?" I asked jokingly, trying to

make light of her advice. She kept a stern look on her face, one that told me this was priceless wisdom.

"You need," she said, lowering her eyes, "those two days to rest."

"I don't know." I shrugged. "I'd probably get sore with all the sex, right?" I laughed.

"You don't have to sleep with them," she said. "You can, but sometimes a hand job will do the trick."

After that first night, Helen and I had dinner often. Like me, she seemed lonely, and I was glad to have someone to hang out with, despite our age difference. Sometimes I'd tag along when she had dinner with old rich men—dentists and surgeons—and anyone else willing to pay the bill for our extravagant feasts. The one time I offered money, Helen just slapped my hand away at the table and told me never to do that again.

"When a woman pays, she's telling the man she doesn't like herself. So why should he?"

When there were just the two of us, Helen spat out her words of wisdom on how to play with men and then take all their money and run. And no matter how brave I got, I never asked the one question burning inside of me: "But does it make you *happy*?"

I can't say now why not. I imagine she would have scoffed at me for asking, not because it was a rude question but because it had an obvious answer. *No*, she wasn't happy, but she probably would've lied and said, "Happiness doesn't matter." And she would've said it with such authority that I might've believed her. Sure, she looked good for her age and there were always men willing to foot the bill for her dinners, but she always came home alone, or else with me.

After dining at Luc's restaurant one night, instead of going home straightaway, Helen said he wanted to have us over for drinks. I hadn't talked much with Luc, except to compliment his cooking and thank him when he didn't charge us.

"He's very interesting," she told me. "I think you'd make a good match."

I looked over at him on the other side of the restaurant, talking to one of his customers, and I started laughing.

"Are you serious? He's too old for me, Helen. And, anyway, I don't find him attractive at all."

"What *is* attractive?" she asked, but it was one of her rhetorical questions, because she called him over right then and told him we'd be happy to join him. I just nodded and smiled. After all, it was the polite thing to do after all those free meals.

"How old are you?" Luc asked, while he rolled us a joint in his living room. He and I were sitting on his love seat. Helen was on the floor beside us.

"She's young," Helen answered for me. "Twenty-three."

He licked the rolling paper and then smiled at me. "Nice," he said. Then I followed his eyes as they traveled down my body. This made me blush. I was wearing a low-cut blouse and I'd felt uncomfortable about it all night.

"That's beautiful," he said, smiling.

"What?" I put my hand to my chest in an attempt to cover my cleavage.

"Your necklace," he clarified, reaching over with one hand to touch a pearl necklace that Helen had let me borrow.

"Oh, it's Helen's," I said, feeling relieved that he wasn't openly talking about my breasts.

I laughed as his hand fell away from my necklace and onto the sofa beside my leg. He was barely touching me, just the edge of his finger, but it was still too much. I was glad when he moved his hand to fetch his lighter from the table and lit the joint. Though I wanted to move to the floor with Helen, I thought it might make me look rude. So I sat there, motionless like a scared deer.

I glanced over at Helen, who had a disappointed expression on her face. She seemed relaxed before, but now annoyed. Maybe I was ruining the mood?

I felt anxious in his house, a dark and messy place, where Asian silk fans hung from the walls like artwork alongside photos of him and his children, who looked to be in their teens.

"How old are your kids?" I asked, taking a small puff on the joint, but not inhaling long enough. I didn't want to get high there because I was afraid it would make me nervous. I already felt nervous, so I took more sips of my champagne.

He didn't want to talk about his kids though. Instead, he talked about Paris, after he noticed my excitement when he mentioned the city. I'd only visited briefly, but it was the number one city on my list of places to live. All the greatest writers had lived there, and clinging to the idea that happiness and success depended upon location, I couldn't think of a more desirable image of myself than as a writer who lived in the city of the greats. London hadn't made me into the big writer, but I had high hopes for the City of Light.

I tried to communicate this desire to him, but it was difficult to convey. I was already feeling a little dizzy from the smoke and champagne, even though I hadn't taken much of the joint myself. All I could say was, "I love Paris," over and over. He didn't try to get more out of me anyway. He didn't seem to be interested in why I loved Paris or anything about me at all, so I asked more questions.

"Why did you come to Hawaii?"

"Things are more relaxed on the island," he said, reaching over to me again. Only this time he didn't touch my necklace. He

touched my bare shoulder. I looked down at my empty champagne glass. "Don't you feel relaxed?" he asked.

Helen got up and yawned loudly. We both looked at her.

"I'm going to lie down," she announced, hurrying out of the
room before I could stop her.

Luc poured me more champagne and smoked the rest of the
joint. At some point, he ran out of things to talk about. That's
when he climbed on top of me and I didn't stop him. He kissed
my mouth, my neck, and my breasts while his hands explored my
body. There was an urgency to his movements and he seemed
hungry, ravenous even. I felt dazed. I knew, for sure, that I didn't
want to be kissing this man, this ex-boyfriend of Helen's who was
older than my own father, but I didn't want to be impolite. The
pot had already taken control of my thoughts, my voice, and my
will. Instead, I ran my fingers through his thinning hair, reclined
back on the couch, and tried to think of something else, my body
working on autopilot.

But I couldn't think of anything else.

Just as I was starting to feel disgusted with him and with myself, something strange happened. There was a shift. An opening.
Suddenly, I felt turned on. I opened my eyes and saw him on top
of me, this old man I didn't know or like, and then I looked over at
the photo of him on the wall with his kids, and I, too, felt like a kid.
Like a little girl who was unsure of herself and didn't know what
else to do but hand herself over to a man, any man, a man who
made her feel like this. Like the schoolgirl who thinks fucking her
teacher after class will score her a better grade on her history test.
Like the attention-hungry teen who tempts her stepdad by leaving
the bathroom door open while she showers, letting suds slip off
her tits while he takes her from behind. Like the bored babysit-
ters. Like the insecure cheerleaders. Like all those young girls in

all those "old and young" category videos that had filled so many hours of my young life.

Giving my body to Luc like this, I was captivated by how erotic and pitiful submission felt. It also became clear to me, in that moment, who Helen really was—she was a madam, a pimp, and I was the new flavor of the island. Excitement and clarity washed over me, and I felt present and rooted in the moment. I felt alive. I felt lit, high, and drunk. I got off on the idea that I was a whore being used, a dirty slut, something to be ashamed of. But this was, of course, only temporary.

Helen walked back in, interrupting the two of us to announce it was time to go home. She seemed unfazed at the sight of us there, a tangle of limbs on the couch, while she waited for Luc to climb off and help me up to stand. I gathered my things and we were soon back on the road after an awkward and rushed good-bye. In the car, Helen told me to be careful and that I should never give it away for free.

"You play your cards right and you can do well for yourself," she told me. "You can travel, buy a house, do whatever the hell you want—just like me."

Sitting in the passenger seat beside her, I stayed silent, watching the dark road ahead. I couldn't see the ocean, but I knew it was just to the other side of the car and down the mountain. Keeping my eyes on the red taillights of some distant car ahead, I felt the erotic thrill of that moment with Luc slowly drain from my system, leaving behind a big black hole.

When I woke up the next day, I avoided Helen as well as I could. Luckily, I had work to distract me from what had happened the night before and how strange I now felt about it. During my shift, a bouquet of red roses arrived for me with a card that read, *Had a great time last night*, signed with Luc's name. I received a text message from Helen asking if I wanted to go on a trip to Waikiki with him, all expenses paid. She said to call her. I excused myself to the bathroom and cried in the stall. I needed to make friends urgently, if only to save myself from people like Helen and Luc and the other rich men she introduced me to. I wasn't ready to cross over into a world of prostitution, but I didn't trust myself enough to say no to the idea, when everything else in my body said yes. The wetness between my legs, my adrenaline coursing through me, my brain serving up images of me on my knees sucking off a strange man for an envelope of cash. I knew that once I made the choice, there was no turning back. What would happen next? What else would I say yes to? I didn't know enough about the real day-to-day lives of sex workers, but I knew that I didn't want to find out.

I wasn't sure what I could do to keep myself safe except to do what I did. Go home with a friendly bartender who worked at my restaurant and convince him, through a flawless blow job, my unrelenting sex drive, and my undivided attention, to be my boyfriend. I needed the structure of a monogamous relationship to keep me from straying too far into the unknown. I needed boundaries.

Greg was a tanned, blue-eyed surfer with a drinking problem. He had recently gotten a DUI and was attending AA meetings, but that didn't stop him from getting blackout drunk every night. For the next few months, we stuck to each other like coconuts on a hula dancer's tits. Because I saw his alcoholism as an obvious flaw and I saw myself as flawed in a number of ways, I tried to imagine that we were compatible.

He never remembered any of our fights. We'd get trashed, try to make love before he got soft from the drinking, get into a fight, fall asleep, and then wake up the next morning to share a giant breakfast. Eggs, bacon, potatoes, Spam, toast, and coffee—we had appetites as big as our problems.

Drinking was an everyday, all-day activity in his life. He'd start with a Bloody Mary, ride the afternoon with cold beers, and end the night with vodka sodas. If we were having a nice dinner, he'd throw in some wine. If we were out at a bar, maybe a few margaritas, and then a vodka soda to cap the night. If we were going to his favorite tequila bar, then a few shots of the best tequila in between Coronas with lime. And then he'd black out. We'd start our days sweet and end them sloppy.

As one month converged into the next, and I still hadn't made any friends, I tried to keep up with Greg's drinking. It helped me excuse his habits of pissing the bed and forgetting to hide other women's clothes in his apartment. So long as he kept me from being lonely or slutty, I was willing to look the other way.[13]

The amount of time Greg and I spent fighting and drinking and trying to recall things came to be this project in my mind of "learning to accept people" for what they were. I didn't want to help Greg or change him; I wanted to love him exactly as he was. After all, if I couldn't love myself completely, then I could at least try to love someone who seemed as broken up inside as I was.

I soon found a way to escape the weirdness of living in Helen's house when my parents decided to buy a vacation condo in

---

13   In her book *Ready to Heal: Breaking Free of Addictive Relationships*, sex-addiction therapist Kelly McDaniel writes that women are "hardwired" for connection. "If connection is not happening, she'll create an illusion of connection. In order to do this, she will develop escape strategies that allow her to adapt to whatever relationship she is currently in." Some common adaptations include being compliant and nice, rather than truthful, lying, abusing substances, or repeatedly choosing unavailable partners.

Maui. My dad's business was booming and I was entrusted with the lucky responsibility of looking after their two-bedroom condo, which had a view of the ocean from the master bedroom and a privacy I couldn't quite get at Helen's.

Not long after I moved into my new place, Greg broke up with me in a drunken rage at a party. He was having a good time, but I was the designated driver, so I couldn't drink. Too many people at the restaurant had gotten DUIs and I was too paranoid to take any chances. While he hung out with his friends, I stewed in the usual panic I found in social situations where alcohol wasn't available, feeling weird and separate from everyone else. When I pulled him aside to tell him I needed to leave and that I would pick him up later, I could tell he was already gone, his eyes unable to focus and his balance wavering. Without lowering his voice, he told me, right there in front of everyone that I should leave. He was tired of me and I wasn't any fun.

"You're so boring!" he yelled.

Humiliated and feeling too many eyes on me, I left the party and returned home, where I masturbated myself to sleep.

I made frantic phone calls to him over the next few days, which turned into weeks, but he didn't want to speak to me, and this made work unbearable when we had to work the same shift. Once again, I was cast off into isolation, my one source of human connection now replaced with that old, familiar sense of emptiness, which could only be answered with my old, familiar set of solutions.

I quit my job at the restaurant and got a new one selling expensive toe rings on the beach. But living on an island as small as Maui makes it virtually impossible to avoid an ex completely. I quickly learned how to divert my eyes, make myself invisible, and flee the discomfort I felt when I ran into him in random places.

Now that I was single, I felt like I had a target on my back.
Men called out to me walking past, approached me to ask for my
name or number, licking their lips while they looked my body up
and down. It was as if a memo had gone around the island letting
everyone know that I wasn't just available, I was desperate. Where
I used to covet a man's interest, feeling empty if I didn't get it, now
the experience only caused me anxiety. I hated being catcalled
and looked at, feeling like I was under a magnifying glass, every
inch of my body open to critique, but I always smiled and played
along, knowing what it could lead to—less time spent alone and
the company of a warm body. As sad and despicable as I felt about
myself, men didn't seem to notice. Or maybe they did notice and
just didn't care. With time, I realized I didn't have to worry about
being alone, because Helen had been right about what she'd
preached many months before. It was possible, if I desired it, to
have multiple "boyfriends"—one for every day of the week.

In LA, I had occasionally experimented with casual sex, and I
always felt guilty afterward. In Hawaii, I took this experimentation
to a new level and I felt guilty all the time. Instead of jumping into
another monogamous relationship, I sought to fill each lonely moment with any body available, no matter the time of day or night.
I accepted invitations from anybody who asked, whether I was
attracted to them or not—home-cooked dinners, restaurant dinners, beers at beachfront bars, wine at fancy hotel bars. A photographer, a construction worker, a landscaper, and a ukulele player.
An art dealer, a drug dealer, a real estate agent, and a poet. I didn't
sleep with all the men I shared drinks and unmemorable conversations with. But the ones I did sleep with I kept on a rotating
basis, so the possibility of me not having sex became a rarity and
a horror.

I flip-flopped constantly between craving my space and hating when I got it. I wanted all the positives of a relationship—the feeling of being desired, the gratification of being touched, the sensation of a man's weight on my body, the potentiality of being loved—but I didn't want all the other baggage. I didn't want the possessiveness of a relationship, wondering where he's at when he's not with me or feeling dependent on one man's dick. I didn't want the buildup to intimacy, the asking of questions, the answering of questions, the getting to know each other's deepest fears and secrets. And most of all, I didn't want the possibility of being hurt by someone because he decided it was time to leave. If a man wanted to leave me now, it was no problem, I told myself, because there would be a new one waiting in the wings. I had no right to get hurt feelings because we weren't together. And neither did they.

Stories about me started floating around the island, and sometimes the men asked if the stories were true. Had I really given a blow job in a parking lot in exchange for a Louis Vuitton purse? Had I really starred in a porn? Though these were lies, I could tell they questioned my denial, and I tried not to let that bother me. Like a mantra, I reminded myself I didn't have to prove anything to them. Nobody could hurt me. I was invincible.

The guy I saw most often was Clay, the six-foot-eight man with crooked teeth and the neck tattoo. I know he was six foot eight, not because I measured him, but because he reminded me about this fact on multiple occasions. *I can't sleep in your bed because it's too small. I'm six foot eight. I don't get drunk that easily because of my size, you know? I'm six foot eight.* Something about him seemed intensely insecure and I think that's what drew me to him. I let him hide behind the size of his body because it made him feel powerful. I nodded and acted surprised every time he announced his measurements because I understood what it was like to hide.

Clay was the one I could count on to make dates and then break them, before showing up high or drunk and horny in the middle of the night, to make me feel like I was his whore, or worse, his last resort. While the other guys sometimes took me out before they fucked me, Clay was silent and self-absorbed and purely sexual. He used me just as much as I used him.

Whenever I finished fucking someone I'd retreat to the bathroom to wash myself, moving slowly, so they'd have some time to think up an excuse for not spending the night. There was a part of me that wanted to be back in a relationship—even the rockiest of them felt safer and more intimate than casual sex, but I mostly wanted to be left alone. Not for too long, of course, just long enough to give myself an orgasm if I hadn't achieved one with the guy, get my porn fix, groom my body, record the night in my journal the way I wanted to remember it, or sleep. When a man did eventually leave, I simmered in conflicted feelings of relief and rejection.

When he stayed, I lied there for hours, unable to relax enough to sleep beside a stranger. I dreaded the idea of spending a day together, having to be sober and make conversation, have him find out who I really was outside of the bedroom or the bar. Even if I saw a man as replaceable, I still feared having him find out the truth—that I was boring and untalented and unlovable. I preferred keeping his perception of me limited to my fuckability and how cool I was about our arrangement. I was edgy, a bit mysterious. Not clingy.

◆

When I noticed four purplish bumps in my groin, I cursed the men I had slept with on the island, trying to recall whether I'd noticed any suspicious bumps on them, but for all the drinking or pot smoking that accompanied these occasions, I couldn't recall a thing.

About a day or so after I noticed these small pea-size bumps around my crotch, I noticed three larger, marble-size bumps in my right armpit. Though they were bigger, they were equally as hard under my fingertip and extremely sensitive. Certain that I hadn't gotten drunk enough to allow a guy to fornicate with my armpit, I immediately headed to the clinic to have my bumps examined.

Within seconds of poking my armpit with her finger, the doctor explained I'd caught staph infection from shaving nicks and ocean water. When she asked if I had them anywhere else, I didn't hesitate from lifting up my skirt, pulling down my bathing suit bottom and showing her my other bumps. Again she confirmed that I was suffering from staph infection, or staph disease as it is casually called, noting that "lots of people get it" and not to worry too much, her face tanned and cheery. She proceeded to cut them open with a scalpel to drain the pus and prescribed Vicodin for the pain.

"Thank God," I said with relief, when it was all over. "At least it's not an STD."

"No, this isn't an STD," she assured me. "But when's the last time you were tested?"

When I shrugged my shoulders, she booked my next appointment.

A few days later, I found out from the doctor that, in addition to staph, I had contracted HPV. The last time I'd been tested was back in college, so I was certain I'd caught the STD in the past year or two from one of the various men I took home, though it wasn't clear from whom. I'd barely used condoms with any of them. Although HPV is one of the most common of the STDs—according to the CDC, about fourteen million people become newly infected each year—I'd never met another girl or guy who'd been diagnosed, so the stigma and seriousness seemed high. I was more disgusted with myself than ever.

To distract myself from feelings of self-hatred, I cut down on the men I saw, smoked a ton of pot, and drank alone while I binged on porn between crying fits. I also fantasized about escaping again, though my funds were now extremely limited. I needed a man to take care of me now, I decided. To not just keep me safe from my promiscuous ways and penchant for loneliness, but to keep me afloat financially. Helen had warned me never to give it away for free, but I couldn't seem to do anything but that.

◆

"Never trust a grown man on a skateboard."

This is something a woman said to me one of my first weeks on the island, when she was giving me a bikini wax. She meant this both literally and figuratively. "The men here are like little boys. The island is good for hooking up, but if you want love, you can't expect to find it from one of the guys here."

"Why not?" I asked.

"There are so many transients—people moving on and off the island all the time—and tourists! So many tourists. Girls looking for an island fling, so they could brag to all their girlfriends back home. You want love? You'll have to find it somewhere else."

Love. This is what I needed now and I wasn't going to find it on the island. I was sure of it. And while I couldn't deny that the problem had more to do with me than my location, the two seemed inseparable. I believed my actions had everything to do with my place of residence because I still clung to the story in my head that London had been pristine. I had been social there and less slutty and happy being alone. I had been confident in myself and interested in the world and productive. Anything that didn't fit the story, like stripping for the photographer or clinging to Anna's male friends, I tried to block.

I would later learn that what I was really caught up in was what addicts call the "geographical cure." There's an adage people love to throw around in recovery—which I still knew nothing about—"Wherever you go, there you are." The illusion that somewhere else would turn me into someone else was so strong that no matter how many times I attempted to escape and ended up in the same place as before, I still believed in the possibility of trying again. The appeal of elsewhere was as powerful in my twenties as it had been when I was a kid in that hotel room with my mom, taking a break from our lives for a while.

Nearing my one-year anniversary on the island, I met Elliot, a filmmaker from New York who was visiting Maui for a few weeks. He was a grown-up. But he wasn't too old, like Luc.

I'm not sure what he saw in me the day he approached my jewelry cart to ask me out. I was convinced someone of his status—someone who lived outside of the Maui bubble—wouldn't notice someone like me. I'm not sure what he continued seeing in me those first few dates, when I silently nodded and acted interested, making little commentary while he enthusiastically divulged details of his interesting and artistic life full of famous people and big success back home. But whatever he saw, it was enough for him to tell me he loved me within weeks of knowing me. It was enough for him to see some kind of promise in me that I desperately wanted to see in myself.

We'd only shared a handful of romantic dinners and had slept together a few times when he asked if I'd consider moving to New York. We were walking along the beach and his question took me by surprise.

"I could introduce you to all the right people," he said. "If you want to be a writer, there's no better place to do it."

Seeing him as my doorway, my ticket, and my savior, the answer was obvious. Of course I would go to New York. I would go to New York and become a successful writer. I would start all over again. An important man was interested in me. This was my chance.

seven

THE NEEDY GIRL

On the surface, my first few weeks in New York were what I'd always wanted them to be. Well, almost. Elliot, who was also from LA, lived in a sun-filled Lower East Side studio near the Tenement Museum. He'd been in the city for over a decade, making indie films, music videos, and some top-rated cable shows. We went to dinner parties and gallery openings and concerts, where I sat backstage as he introduced me to people I recognized from television. I tried to hold myself confidently as I shook their hands and said hello, hoping they didn't notice my sweaty palm. But I could never keep from feeling starstruck and inferior. I often excused myself for bathroom breaks, just to sit in the stall and catch my breath. His world was exciting. I felt uncomfortable, misplaced.

Growing up in LA, I felt so close to the action yet so far away. Driving through Hollywood, only twenty minutes from my painfully mediocre home in Montebello, the glamour of that place was undeniable and I was drawn to it, but I knew it wasn't for me. As a child, watching television with my mom in bed, it was clear to me that there were two worlds that rarely mixed: us and them. I felt like an imposter on Elliot's big, beautiful stage.

During those first few weeks, he sat me down to give me a heartfelt talk about how I didn't have to worry about "a thing." What he meant was the rent: I could devote all my time to writing, he said, sheltered by his multicolored walls strewn with photographs of stars he'd worked with and awards he'd won—souvenirs of his important work.

His last project, a reality show, had paid him well enough that we could live pretty luxuriously; we hired a maid, sent our laundry out, had our groceries delivered, bought thirty-day MetroCards, saw lots of concerts, and slept until noon. We took his dog to the dog park, ate brunch in the trendiest cafés, and lazily read the paper. The Arts and Real Estate sections were his; I took Comics and Travel. He taught me that Manhattan was like a grid, showed me what neighborhoods I could explore at night and which I should avoid. It didn't matter much because I didn't want to explore anything without him. I told myself that's what love was. That's how love should always be.

But as time passed, I came to dread, with even more intensity than before, those moments when Elliot introduced me to yet another friend or acquaintance. Mostly, I dreaded that common yet terrifying question: "So, Erica, what do you do?" This kind of question had never really stumped me before, even when I was just waitressing or working retail, but there was something infinitely more intimidating about all these new people asking. And their inquiries would continue to haunt me throughout the entirety of our relationship, making me feel like I was in way over my head. That I had to try harder. That I had to become better than I was.

After a tense laugh, the answer I'd give for the next few months whenever I'd meet someone new was: "Well, I just got to New York, so I'm still figuring it out." Then I'd chug my drink if I had one, escape to the bathroom, or smile in humiliation when Elliot tried to overcompensate by explaining, "Well, Erica's a writer . . . ," which felt like a total lie. He'd never even read anything that I'd written.

Worse, as soon as it sunk in that I was cohabitating with someone, my usual habits and the secrecy that surrounded them became all the more intense. In the morning, Elliot would grab his big blue book and a banana, kiss me good-bye, and head off to his AA meeting—he'd been sober for five years—while I feigned sleepiness, and I'd wait fifteen minutes to make sure he was gone for good so I could start my day. I'd get up, throw on some clothes, walk his dog a quick lap around the block, and then race her back up our five flights of stairs to obsessively groom my body and masturbate before he got home.

My relationship with Elliot was the first one that did not revolve around sex. This would become a huge problem for me. In fact, it was a problem from the start, although I was careful not to mention it often because I feared what his reaction might be. We had sex maybe once or twice a week, which in retrospect isn't that bad, and he assured me that this was normal for a man nearly forty, but it never felt like enough. On top of that, I had trouble relaxing enough to actually enjoy myself so that when it was over, I felt desperately dissatisfied and depressed.

Part of the reason I could not relax, even though I usually felt sex was the most promising thing I had to offer a man, was because of his colorful past. I had picked up on the fact that he had dated many actresses from his films, most of whom I admired. One had even been nominated for an Oscar, a familiar presence on magazine covers. This led me to feel hopelessly inadequate in comparison and avoid the magazine aisles at the supermarket. I couldn't help from wondering—why had he gone from someone like her to someone like me? What did I have to offer?

It wasn't just his romantic past that made me feel inadequate. He had done so much with his life already—went to grad school, lived in Paris, had magazine articles written about him—and I doubted I'd ever catch up. It didn't matter that I was only twenty-four years old and had time to accomplish my own dreams; I just couldn't figure out which dream to accomplish first and how to do it fast enough before he grew tired of me and kicked me out of his glitzy life.

Even though he didn't ask me for any money, I tried to find a job right away, but my résumé didn't land me any of the cool writing or publishing jobs I coveted and applied to in bulk. I thought about waitressing again, but that felt like a tragic step backward. So I tried to focus my efforts on being domestic, even though I burned every meal I tried to cook. I got myself a credit card and bought him gifts now and then, even though he assured me that I needn't waste my money.

Without the usual crutch of sex filling most of our time together, I became self-conscious about the most miniscule things. Did he like the clothes I wore? Did I bring up interesting conversation topics? Does he like the books I read? I quieted these fears by studying pictures of his famous ex-girlfriends online and charging new clothes to my credit card, scouring news sites and celebrity gossip blogs to have new things to talk about all the time, and reading only the books I found on his bookshelf or those he recommended.

When I look back now, I can't say that we had much in common besides wanting to create art for a living. We were both dissatisfied with what we'd done with our lives thus far, although this confused me because, in my eyes, he'd done so much. But one of the reasons he sought sobriety was because he felt that he had allowed his addictions to get in the way of his career at various points—pissing off all the wrong people, taking too long to get some projects off the ground—and now he wanted to be sure that he made up for any lost time.

We had little to talk about beyond whatever project he was dreaming up next, or how old projects had played out, tidbits of gossip about people he knew or wanted to know. The rest of the time, we shared a lot of uncomfortable silence. My brain wasn't silent though. Insults followed me around all day. *You're boring him! Say something funny! Say something interesting! Make him love you!*

I was as flattered as I was confused when, months in, Elliot asked me to marry him. I thought back over our brief time together and how uncomfortable I still felt around him, and I told myself a lie: *As soon as we're married, I'll feel better.*

We flew back to LA to share the news with our families and even though most of them congratulated us with best wishes, I will never forget the look on my mom's face. She gave me a feeble smile as she pulled me close and tightly squeezed. "Congratulations, baby," she said softly. "I hope you're happy." I knew, all too well, when she pitied me.

While Elliot watched sports with my dad, I talked incessantly to her and my sister until my throat hurt about how great my life was in New York. I mentioned all the famous people I'd met, the cool parties, and Elliot's upcoming projects.

"And what are you working on?" she asked. "Are you writing much?"

My face went hot, but I tried to shrug it off. "I'm just happy living right now."

What did she know, anyway? My life was fabulous. Wasn't it?

On that trip, although we spent that afternoon at my parents' house, we spent most of our time at Elliot's family's house in Santa Monica, where he said he felt more comfortable. His AA meetings were there, his friends were there, he slept better there . . . the list went on and on. I felt guilty not spending more time with my parents, whom I hadn't seen in what felt like forever, but I would do anything Elliot said at that point. His comfort was my priority.

His parents' house was gorgeous—three stories, a beautiful pool and greenhouse, artwork and antiques. His mother had an eye for art and design, so the house was impeccably decorated. And she was gorgeous too, with black, shiny hair, interesting jewelry, and a face free of wrinkles.

In the mornings, she served us lox, bagels, coffee, and fresh fruit in her immaculately white kitchen. Sitting across from her at the table, I felt too casual in my pajamas, even though Elliot wore his. She carried herself elegantly in crisp blouses and perfectly applied lipstick and ate her food in tiny bites. She talked about art and gardening and theater and politics, and I didn't know what to say, so I just nodded. I wondered if she got along better with Elliot's exes and if she was as confused as I was about why he'd settled on me. I found being around her and the rest of his family as intimidating as any of the social situations I'd experienced over the last few months. That's when it dawned on me that it didn't really matter whether the people Elliot knew were famous, because his mother clearly wasn't and she still scared the hell out of me.

◆

When we returned to New York engaged, Elliot landed a few new jobs, some of which took him out of state. I landed my own jobs— working at a boutique that sold baby clothes and tutoring a couple of rich kids on the Upper East Side. With time to myself, instead of feeling more secure and independent, I now felt suspicious all day about what Elliot was doing without me. I was convinced that it was only a matter of time before he left me for one of the hotter, younger, more talented actresses on set. And how could I blame him?

I started reading his journals when he was away, loading up on details about his fabulous life before me and all the famous women he'd slept with. I also found entries he'd written about me, some of them sweet and full of praise, but some far less flattering. One entry detailed his "obsession" with my body hair, which I thought I had kept under meticulous control at this point in my life. In the entry, he seemed to be facing a vicious mental struggle with fully accepting my physical flaws, even though he knew love was supposed to "go deeper." Suddenly, it made sense to me why we didn't have much sex and why it was over so quickly when we did. He was disgusted with me. Not only was I boring and untalented—I was ugly too.

Humiliated, I called him up and unleashed fury. But instead of apologizing for what he wrote and building me back up with compliments like I wanted him to, or *needed* him to, he reacted with anger. He couldn't get past the fact that I had disrespected his boundaries by reading his journal. His disappointment in me was yet another harsh blow to my self-esteem.

So I decided I would fix myself. I'd be better at hair removal, yes, but I'd also be better at everything else in my life. Over the next few months, while Elliot worked more and we talked about the wedding less, I went on a spree of self-help trials. I committed to yoga three times a week, trying to settle my racing mind through a series of sun salutations. I had little hope for my mind, which seemed a mess, setting my hopes on a tight ass at the very least, but then I found a Buddhist temple for group meditation, where monks chanted and I dutifully clenched my eyelids tight, praying,

praying for some divine intervention to make me into someone else before I lost it all. I went to Al-Anon meetings, hoping that the least I could do was try to understand Elliot's addiction, but I only wished the minutes away. I enrolled in an art class on the Lower East Side, mashing paint and canvas together into concoctions I hated and threw away after class. And I applied to grad schools for writing across the city, the most prestigious ones as well as the ones I'd never heard about. I didn't care which one I got into, I just needed someone to validate my voice—the voice I'd only ever reserved for the page.

I was impatient. I wanted change and I wanted it now. The problem was that I didn't know how to replace my old habits and skills to support the new ones. Sure, I wasn't sleeping around—I was barely sleeping with Elliot—but there was still the porn, now accessible via smartphone across endlessly updated websites, still the disgust with myself, still the shame.

And my motivations for changing continued to revolve around achieving the same results—losing myself in some man's affection and approval, in the sensations between my legs. What I couldn't figure out was how to calmly desire something new. Something wildly different from what had stopped serving me long ago. Or perhaps had never served me at all.

Elliot said he was impressed with all my new interests, yet the space between us swelled. Sex became even more infrequent, and while I usually waited for him to make the first move, now I bravely initiated, only to be rejected. My need for affection became unbearable. If I brought up the wedding, he would tell me he was busy. If he felt an argument bubbling up, he'd excuse himself from my presence and head to yet another AA meeting. I felt hopelessly abandoned and utterly unworthy.

When he was out of the house, I found myself crossing more

boundaries. Checking his email for evidence of his infidelities, digging through the trash can and his pockets for condoms or suspicious receipts, and reading more of his journals. He wasn't fucking me—so who *was* he fucking? I questioned his whereabouts all the time and didn't believe anything he told me. He began to sigh at me more than he smiled at me. When I brought up the lack of sex one afternoon, figuring it was the one thing I could fix if I tried my hardest, he fired back, "Have you wondered if you might be a sex addict? I can't keep up with you. Look into Sex and Love Addicts Anonymous meetings." Then he said he was going to a meeting. Furious, I followed him to the door. I was so full of rage I wanted to shove him, but I shouted at him instead.

"I'm not a sex addict, asshole! You just don't fuck me enough!"

He slammed the door shut.

Instead of going to SLAA meetings like he suggested, fearing I'd be the only woman there, I went to Co-Dependents Anonymous meetings (CoDA). Together, with a small group of people, I shared my relationship fears in a church basement. I hadn't talked at any of the Al-Anon meetings and I hadn't listened much there either. CoDA felt a lot more like home. While most people talked about their parental issues, I could relate to the general feeling of neediness and pain that overshadowed the room, and I found the vulnerability refreshing.

After one of these meetings, a woman with platinum-blond hair and bright pink lipstick approached me and said, "I listened to your share and I have to say, it really sounds like you could use SLAA meetings." She gave me a small piece of paper with an address scrawled out. I thanked her and threw the paper away as soon as I was outside. I had no interest in examining my relationship with sex and I was afraid going to SLAA would require abstinence. The thought was horrifying.

I found a therapist I could barely afford. For $150 an hour, I sat in a dim office near Union Square and resented this curly-haired woman with a Long Island accent for her obligatory nods and "tell me mores" while I tiptoed around my life history and tried to prove to her how smart and interesting I was. At our first meeting, I talked about my travels and how great my parents were and how talented my fiancé was. When she pushed for more, I shrugged my shoulders defiantly, feeling terrified of revealing too much and being assessed as a crazy person.

"Then what do you want to work on, Erica?" she asked. "How can I help?"

"I'm not sure," I said, staring down at my hands. I hoped she couldn't see them shaking. "I'm just not feeling . . ." I paused, feeling uncertain of what I wanted to feel. "I guess I'm not feeling happy."

Over time, crumbs fell from my mouth. I told her about how I couldn't stop reading his journal, how we weren't having sex, how I obsessed about his past and about my body, and how I was anxious and insecure around everybody, including him. She jotted down notes and I even resented her for that.

Then, surprisingly, at the start of one of our sessions, she announced that she had something to tell me. Usually our meetings began in awkward silence until I brought up a random topic, but on this day, she looked driven and possibly excited.

"I have a diagnosis," she said.

It was the first time I felt pleased to be in therapy. Not even a year in and already an explanation? I suddenly noticed that her Long Island accent had a comforting quality to it and her curly hair softened her face. I felt bad for having thought less of her and considered my money well spent.

I had the fourth most common disorder in America, she said. I shrugged off my lack of uniqueness and embraced the word *disor-der. Finally, a name for this. A name for whatever this is.*

"Obsessive Compulsive Disorder. OCD."

It was not what I was expecting.

"No, not the kind who counts," she said. "No, not the type who can't stop washing his hands." She explained that my obsessions and habits could be cured. Those racing thoughts about Elliot in bed with his ex-girlfriends? We could fix that. Those hours spent obsessing about my hair follicles? No big deal. My sexual crav-ings? No longer my problem.

She advised me to see my physician because she had an idea that might help. Zoloft. I knew the name—images of a big, doughy, depressed bubble flopping around in television ads came to mind while she enthusiastically went on about how versatile the drug was. How it would also help those social problems I'd mentioned to her and the extra irritability I felt around my period. Zoloft would help soften the mood swings, help me to remain balanced, and lead me to a calmer and more productive sort of life. I won-dered if my initial glee was what born-again Christians felt. Zoloft sounded like my savior, and I wanted to start anew.

A couple of days later I visited my physician, Dr. K, who was an Eastern European man with kind eyes. Sitting on the paper sheet of the examining table, I gave highlights of my predicament. He nodded sympathetically, jotting down notes on his pad of paper while he murmured, "I understand," over and over, but within minutes of explaining my situation and inquiring about Zoloft, Dr. K agreed that a pill would be my savior. Of course I'd only named "anxiety" as the culprit in my life, figuring jealousy and journal reading might've led to more medications than I wanted to try. He gave me a "medium-size dose" and I took the pills, hoping that I'd finally found my cure.

Two weeks passed before I felt a noticeable difference. Besides lethargy, the biggest change was that I could no longer reach orgasm. I watched the type of porn that usually got me off but to no success. Then I watched harder clips and those didn't work either. Reaching climax was suddenly impossible.

I returned to Dr. K and told him what was happening. He smiled, said he understood, but he didn't jot any notes down this time. Five minutes of explanation was enough for him to assign a new remedy: Xanax. Elliot didn't agree with this when he caught me popping the pills, and neither did my therapist, who questioned Dr. K's credibility immediately. But I didn't care, because in less than an hour after popping Xanax, I experienced noticeable results. Xanax and Zoloft, when used together, provided an overall sense of blissful numbness.[14] I didn't care if I couldn't climax or if Elliot was thinking about fucking somebody else or if I was the ugliest woman in the world. I didn't care about anything.

Over the next couple of months, Elliot spent more time out of the apartment, I stopped wearing the engagement ring, and we acted more like distant roommates than lovers, even though we still slept in the same bed—each of us crunched up on our respec-

---

14   Drugs have played and continue to play a role in treating compulsive sexual behaviors, as outlined in a 2006 study by Dr. Timothy W. Fong called "Understanding and Managing Compulsive Sexual Behaviors." There are no US FDA-approved medications for compulsive sexual behaviors, but various classes have been tried, including antidepressants, mood stabilizers, antipsychotics, and even antiandrogens. Research found that while SSRIs, like Zoloft, may decrease the urges/craving and preoccupation associated with sexual addiction, attempting to use SSRIs to create sexual dysfunction through their side-effect profile, and thus reduce compulsive sexual behaviors, does not appear to be effective.

tive sides. In a positive turn of events, one of the more prestigious grad schools I'd applied to accepted me into their writing program. I'd be starting in the fall, finally taking my work seriously enough, though at a $50,000 yearly price tag. Adding "MFA in progress" to my résumé also helped me land my first "real" job as a copywriter at a digital marketing agency in Midtown.

When I worked up the courage to mention to Elliot that I was thinking of moving out, he didn't try to talk me out of it. Instead, he sighed with relief. He even offered to leave the apartment for a few weeks so I could sort out my things and find a new place.

I moved to Brooklyn, and we never spoke again.

◆

What happened next should have been enough to keep me happy—had I only been ready for happiness.

First, I weaned myself off my meds and started to wake up from the slumber of numbness. I won't say it was easy having to feel all my feelings again, and there were definitely low points that made me question my sanity, but nothing positive had come out of being medicated, and I knew that.

I excelled in my writing program despite envying all my classmates for their talents. I acted as I often had in social situations— I kept to myself and obsessed about my inferiority, wondering when they'd all figure out I was a fraud and I didn't know what the hell I was doing. It didn't matter that I'd been accepted into the program. It wasn't enough validation. My classmates appeared confident and far more intelligent than I, and I could already envision their book deals materializing before the next semester arrived. Still, I earned praise and helpful advice from my professors. I wrote a lot about body hair and the shame I felt around my body. I wrote about feeling isolated. I wrote about Elliot and other men.

My details were sparse though, and I was afraid to be completely open and vulnerable, leaving my professors to constantly push for more and countless journal and magazine editors to reject my submissions.

I befriended chatty women from my office job and we went out often, sharing laughs and secrets over glasses of wine and over-priced appetizers. Just as in my younger years, I found socializing easy when I had a drink in my hand and nasty words to say about people I didn't know that well. Gossip and drink are the currency of insecure girls trying desperately to connect.

I reconnected with one of my younger female cousins, Sunny, and she moved into my Brooklyn apartment from California. We made up for lost time over joints, thrift-store hunting, and *Curb Your Enthusiasm* bingeing.

And though not much time had passed since Elliot—a little over a month—I found myself in a new relationship with a dark-eyed man named Noah. He was tall and soft-spoken, and never before had I met someone who seemed so entirely content with his life. During the day he worked at an investment firm. At night, he played the drums in a rock band at dingy bars across the city.

"Is that your big dream?" I asked. "To be a rock star?"

"Nah," he said, smiling. "I'm happy just doing gigs here and there."

One of my coworkers had introduced us at a bar—they had mutual friends—and we quickly abandoned the group for a corner where we could talk alone. I could tell he was shy by the way he avoided eye contact as he told me about his childhood in upstate New York, how he abandoned the violin for the drums, why he thought Bruce Springsteen was the greatest living artist on earth. Even when he asked for my phone number, he stared at the bottle of beer in his hands instead of me.

I was relieved to jump into a new relationship. It was the easi-
est way to move on from the past and resist feeling guilty about any
of my actions. But while Noah was gentle, affectionate, and treated
me like gold, my response was to treat him like shit.

His contentedness with life annoyed me. *Why didn't he try
harder to make his music his career? Could he really be happy at his
job? Did he seriously want to live in New York forever? How could
he not want to see the world?*

I constantly reminded myself that I was superior to Noah in all
ways—I was better educated, read more books, had traveled more,
didn't smoke as much pot, was better looking and far more sexually experienced. I didn't always point out these things, but when
I'd had a few drinks, I would mock him all night, pick fights with
him, and have jealous fits. *Are you checking out that girl? Who did
you have lunch with? Why didn't you pick up your phone earlier?*
When I awoke sober, my mouth spewed apologies and I tried to
make up for whatever wrath I'd unleashed on him through sex,
which we were thankfully having plenty of. I imagine this was the
only reason he stuck around as long as he did.

It's not that I didn't like him. It's that I liked him too much. I
liked that it took him three dates to kiss me. I liked that we waited
a whole month before we had sex, even though I'd invited him
back to my place on our very first date. I liked the music he played
in his band—the way he'd bang on the drums like he was banging
through the earth to reach its core. I liked the stories he told, the
way his eyes widened and his voice boomed on the exciting bits.
I liked the way he talked to his mother, the loyalty he had with his
friends, his complete and utter trustworthiness. And how could
I not like the way he brought me coffee and warm croissants in
bed, or the way he looked at me—like I was precious, a gift, something to be studied? I couldn't bear to think of how much it would

hurt to actually let myself love him if I was only going to lose him in the end. The situation with Elliot had confirmed that I should be wary of all relationships, especially ones that seemed to be the real deal. So I placed myself up on a pedestal and told myself that he was just a temporary prop in my life. Someone to fill the time until the next thing came along, whether that thing would be yet another new city to become infatuated with or a new man.

We carried on with our relationship and I grew fonder the more I tried not to. He took me on trips upstate to his parents' house in the Hudson Valley, where we picked apples and played board games. To Philadelphia, where his brother lived. To rock concerts and art galleries and on weekend adventures to places he knew I'd love—Coney Island, Emily Dickinson's house, Tanglewood. I took him to LA, drove him up the coast to see the cliffs in Malibu and the wineries in Santa Barbara. We gambled alongside my parents in Las Vegas and danced at my cousin's wedding in Tennessee. We talked about what it would be like if we got married. Then we stopped saying "if." Of course we'd get married.

But all along, I developed various escape routes just in case we didn't work out. I didn't tell him (because it would've made me a hypocrite with all the jealous rules I held him to), but I reconnected with numerous ex-lovers online—men in LA and Hawaii and Europe whom I kept as backup plans for when things went south. I binged on porn whenever he wasn't around, sent naked photos of myself to people on Craigslist, and fantasized about sleeping with everyone—his friends, my colleagues, his roommates, my neighbors. The only reason I didn't escape right away—leave him before he left me—was because I'd paid so much money for grad school that I had to at least see it to the end.

When I went out with friends and coworkers, I flirted with anyone who looked my way. One evening I joined two of my colleagues at a client event. We were handling the marketing for a trendy boutique hotel in Chelsea, and all the head honchos were there letting loose on the rooftop bar. We ordered drinks and made polite talk with our new clients, careful not to bring up work to kill their buzz, but also careful not to get too casual and mess up our business deal. At some point in the night, I found myself in a conversation with the owner of the hotel, an older Egyptian man in an expensive suit. I don't remember what we were talking about, but I do remember how close his face was to mine and that he smelled like smoke and Scotch. I was the one who suggested he give me a tour of the hotel's best room.

"It'll help me get a better idea of what to write when I'm working on the website," I said to him.

I remember the puzzled looks on my coworkers' faces and the knowing smiles of our clients as I told them all I'd be right back and exited the bar with the owner. He didn't take me to the best room as I requested. He took me to the nearest room to the bar and pulled me onto the bed with him. I laughed and playfully pushed him away as I got back on my feet, a little dizzy now as I pretended to check out the room and act professional.

"Come back," he said, patting the bed.

"What do I get in return though?" I asked, propping one foot up on the bed and spreading my legs so he could see up my skirt.

"You want money?" He dug into his pocket.

I thought about it, but I knew that wasn't it. I didn't want money, I wanted to hurt someone—in this case, Noah—and I wanted to hurt myself in the process. I wanted to destroy the good things in my life because I didn't deserve anything good. I deserved all that was sickening and shameful. But not tonight. Not yet.

"This isn't the best room," I said. "Let's go back to the party." And so we did.

It would take three years with Noah in New York—years I spent trying not to love him, drinking too much, working too much, and fighting too much—before I'd let the multiple drinks and the voice in my head urge me to finally cross those lines and destroy everything.

After graduating from the MFA program, I treated myself to a trip back to Hawaii. While there, I met up with one of my ex-lovers, a Colombian waiter named Andres whom I used to fuck. We drank tequila shots and danced together to Marvin Gaye songs playing on the jukebox of some dive bar and I convinced myself through a series of clichés—*You only live once!*—to let him come home with me and come all over me. I told myself that nobody had to know. The adrenaline racing through my body made me feel invincible at the time. And the shame I felt afterward was even better.

When I returned to New York, I couldn't look Noah in the eyes without hating myself. No longer was I on the pedestal. He was. That couldn't work either. In some crazy stroke of luck, I wrote up a lengthy proposal for my boss, requesting that I keep my position and salary but be allowed to work remotely—from Europe, Hawaii, wherever I wanted. He accepted. Instead of owning up to my actions with Noah and communicating my fears and my mistakes so we could actually build something together, I scurried away like a child who broke her mother's finest china, and bought a one-way ticket to Paris.

When I told him I was leaving, that I needed to go "find myself," Noah was crushed. I remember him pulling me close to him on his bed and sobbing into my neck so that my hair and the mattress became wet with tears.

"I feel like I'm losing my best friend," he murmured.

You deserve so much more, I thought.

◆

For a few months I attempted to satisfy my lofty dreams, scribbling in my notebook next to glasses of red wine in all the cafés Hemingway used to love, taking long walks along the Seine and spending hours gawking at art in all the best museums. I also spent some time in Barcelona, but I was less into my writing there and more into the music on the streets and what felt like one endless party. And while I wrote here and there and enjoyed myself when I wasn't writing copy for my job back in New York, I couldn't get Noah off my mind or the fear that I'd made a terrible mistake—the kind of mistake you don't shake, not for years, perhaps ever.

To silence this fear, I slept with whoever approached me during my travels. Whoever showed the slightest interest. It almost felt like my time in Hawaii, only worse, because now I was aware. I knew I should be different by now. Nothing satisfied me—not the attention of these men, or the orgasms they gave me, or the views from their bedroom windows. I feared I'd never be satisfied.

At one particularly low moment, I found myself wandering the streets of some unfamiliar Paris suburb I didn't know the name of, trying to find a taxi at three in the morning. My clothes were torn in odd places and I was shivering because I'd left my sweater at the apartment of some French college kid who'd waited on me in a restaurant earlier that evening. I'd holed up in that restaurant all night, pretending to be content and busy with my notebook after I'd long finished my meal, because he'd invited me home with him after his shift. Ordering one glass of wine after another, I couldn't wait to be underneath him in bed, my brain shut off, my body useful again. When we made it there, I let him use my body however he wanted to, without protest. He threw me on the bed, literally ripped my clothes off, and fucked me so hard that when I finally made it home, I had to throw my underwear and tights away because of all the blood. After he came, he walked me to his front door and told me taxis weren't hard to find, before slapping me on the ass and sending me on my way. I threw up the next morning, either because of the wine or disgust, or both.

◆

Unsure of what to do next, I left Europe and returned to Hawaii with two suitcases and my emptiness in tow.

The first thing I did was meet up with the Colombian guy I took home when I was with Noah, as if to justify my decision that night and finally defuse the regret I still felt about it. I thought to myself that if we fell in love and lived happily ever after, then having broken my relationship wasn't a mistake.

But our short and intense attempt at a relationship couldn't have been more different from what I had with Noah, and it only made me miss him more. Still, I tried to force the thing, even when it quickly became clear to me that this thing was all about sex and nothing more meaningful than that.

Andres owned a huge beach house in Maui and another huge beach house in Mexico. He traveled to South America often to take ayahuasca and DMT in the Amazon, bringing mysterious crates home with him. I thought maybe he inherited his money, since it seemed unlikely that serving food a few hours a week could amount to what he had. But after some pushing I discovered that he was only a waiter on paper. He had a series of shady side businesses, one of which was running a live-cam porn site out of his house in Mexico.

He hated revealing this information to me, not because he didn't want me to worry or to judge him, but because he didn't want me to report some of his side dealings if things didn't work out between us. And, after about a month, it was clear things weren't working out between us. He was relentlessly jealous about my past and demanded to know details of my whereabouts whenever I wasn't with him. He didn't believe anything I told him, even when I was clear about not having any other friends on the island besides him—that all the people I had known years ago had left.

He was just as demanding in the bedroom, and his fantasies were extreme. "We could make good money off your slutty little mouth," he'd say, his legs trembling, both hands fastened to my skull, motioning the blow job just the way he liked it—hard and fast. The favorite of his fantasies was thinking about pimping me out. "You'll just get on your knees when I say and I'll get all these guys to line up and give you their cocks. Would you like that? WOULD YOU?"

I'd hum an "Uh-huh," since I obviously couldn't answer him back. My compliance made him both resent me and desire me. He came as soon as I gave him that risky answer he both wanted and hated to hear. "Fucking whore," he'd call out as I swallowed with a harsh gulp. Spitting wasn't allowed here. It meant I didn't really like him.

Sex with him was painful. Both physically and emotionally. There was a lot of choking, slapping, and hair pulling involved, and he'd always find a way to verbally demean me. He loved saying that my only purpose in life was to suck his cock. The only worth I had was in my pussy. Most of the things he said were things that I had thought before, but nobody had ever spoken them aloud like this. I was always wet when I was with him and wet when I was away from him, thinking about him. But there was little time for anything else. And I wasn't interested in anything else anyway. I wanted only him, and he knew how to keep me busy.

When we were together, it was impossible not to have sex.

He'd pull his cock out when he was driving. After we finished having dinner at a restaurant. In the back of some bar. I'd undress for him—slowly and seductively, just the way he liked it—and spin around so he could inspect every crevice before he had me however he wanted me. His appetite was even more incessant than mine, and although I often emerged bruised and exhausted, I continued to gorge myself on him. Even though I hated the fact that he ran porn sites and it was obvious to me that I wasn't the only person he was sleeping with, I continued spending all my time with him, becoming further entangled with every orgasm.

My own mind filled with fantasies of him and his live-cam girls back in Mexico. We watched a ton of porn when we had sex, and his favorite scenes were from casting-call couches—porn site CEOs trying out their new eighteen-year-old merchandise for all the world to see. I wondered if this was the sort of thing Andres did when he went back to Mexico and hired new girls. The thought enraged and excited me at once. I was hooked on feeling like just another one of his cam girls. Another one of his used-up sluts.

I was not hooked on the time we spent outside of the bedroom—trying to make conversation, eat meals together, cultivate a relationship. Neither of us seemed willing to try. I was also annoyed by his mistrust in me, which gave me a whole new perspective on how I'd treated men in my previous relationships. Jealousy wasn't sexy. I got that now.

Little by little, I inched away from him, which was a lot easier to do when I met Oliver, an English guy who hired me for some freelance writing. Oliver was entirely different from Andres—much more polite and a bit nervous around me—and I found this disparity refreshing.

I told Oliver and Andres about each other right away because

I was in no mood to cheat on Andres after how things had ended with Noah. Andres wasn't having it.

"He's just a friend," I insisted. "I make friends with guys easier than girls!"

"Yeah, because they want to fuck you, you idiot," he shot back.

But this didn't stop me. Although I wasn't particularly attracted to Oliver, I liked spending time with him more than I did with Andres because we actually had things to talk about. He was well-read and well-traveled and didn't try to get me into bed right away, like most of the guys I'd met lately.

It didn't take long for the threats to begin. Even though they hadn't met, Andres said he'd find Oliver and make him pay for driving the two of us apart. And then he'd make me pay. Then my family. I tried not to take anything too seriously. I'd been a jealous girlfriend before and had made my fair share of insane threats. But when one fight ended with him throwing me up against a wall, I decided we had to end things. I made my own threats so he'd back off, and went running into the arms of Oliver.

For a few months, I attempted again to force a relationship that didn't exactly work. Although Oliver and I had a good rapport and he was respectful and kind, I simply wasn't romantically interested, even though my body said otherwise. I just didn't want to be alone. To help quiet my mind, I gulped down margaritas and spent most of my time in his bed, hoping that, in time, my heart would eventually catch up.

One night, we decided to take ecstasy together, a drug I'd always been curious about but had been too scared to try. I told him about my fears of overdosing, but he assured me we'd be safe.

"It's the best drug I've ever taken," he said. "Believe me, you'll have an amazing time."

Amazing was an understatement. Some time after taking it, I

remember sinking back into his couch and feeling something I had not felt in years. A complete and utter sense of peace. I didn't feel the need to say or do anything, even when he asked if I wanted to dance with him on the other side of the room or cuddle. I just smiled and shook my head at him, not feeling like I had to give an explanation. Where my mind was usually racing about what to say next or if we should have sex again, I found comfort in silence. In fact, I didn't want to have sex at all, which was strange, because I'd imagined an ecstasy trip to make me hornier than I'd ever been. It was like looking through a window and seeing this whole new beautiful world where pleasure existed without my need to do anything. Just breathing was satisfying enough.

"Now is the time you should probably talk about what happened to you," he said, grabbing my hands and bringing me to my feet.

"What do you mean?" I asked. I felt myself smiling at him with such uncontrollable enthusiasm. "Sorry, I can't stop smiling."

"Don't apologize for that," he said, laughing. "But I mean, is anything coming up for you? Is there anything that hurts? Anything you need to work through?"

I kept smiling, but I was confused. I'd imagined ecstasy to be all about sucking on lollipops and dancing to techno, but he seemed to want to go deeper.

"Trust me," he said. "Someone once did this for me and it changed my life."

Suddenly, he looked like a therapist, but I felt open, so I nodded and began.

I started talking about when I was a kid—all the way back to twelve years old, when I got that back brace and my baby sister was still brand-new and everyone was too busy to help me. I told him how excluded I felt, how scary it was to be alone, how scary it all still was. Words rolled out of me in waves like I'd been holding them in for years. And the funny thing is that it didn't bring me down. It felt like exactly the thing I needed to be talking about. It was important and true and such a relief to say out loud. And all along, he held me through it, listening and nodding and encouraging me to say more.

Afterward, as if to celebrate my purge, we went to the beach across the street from his apartment building. Staring up at the stars, I thought for a moment, *This is what life's supposed to feel like.* And I felt deserving and worthy.

The downside is that, hours later, I crashed hard, harder than I had read about online, and I felt lower than I'd ever felt. Shattered and alone. Even though Oliver was right beside me, experiencing his own comedown, I couldn't have felt further from him. I looked at him and had a flashback of what I'd told him and felt so exposed and broken and terrible about myself and not equipped to handle it. Before I could burst into tears from humiliation, I rushed home and crawled into bed, where I stayed for weeks, making up excuses to skip work and ignoring his phone calls. Hours were whisked away, where I cried and drank and masturbated, trying to pick myself up to no avail. It felt like I'd opened up a deep wound and couldn't stitch it back up. The only solution I could come up with was to leave again.

eight

THE CURIOUS GIRL

With my thirtieth birthday coming up in the summer of 2012, soul-searching in a sacred land seemed an appropriate decision. To make a celebration out of it, I invited along my cousin Sunny, whom I'd lived with in New York, and together we rented a quaint villa in the rice paddies of Ubud, Bali, just like Elizabeth Gilbert did in *Eat Pray Love*.

In the first week we did all the touristy things: feed bananas to mischievous monkeys at the Monkey Forest; taste the most expensive coffee in the world, Kopi Luwak, made from the feces of the Asian palm civet; applaud fire dancers; tour the rice terraces; and indulge in $10 massages every day. We spent my birthday at a cremation ceremony, which was a far cry from the dull and depressing processions of Western burials. There was a parade in the street, colorful outfits, gong music, children playing—truly a celebration. And there was something beautiful in welcoming another year of life while someone was bidding farewell to their own in such spectacular fashion.

It was also refreshing to spend so much time with Sunny, whom

I had always been fond of but usually only in between my day-to-day romantic dramas. She reminded me of happy moments I'd long forgotten from childhood—playing hide-and-go-seek with all the boys in the family and all those trips we made together as kids, from the snowy slopes of Big Bear to the sun-kissed beaches of San Diego. I'd spent so much time obsessing about this guy and that guy, I'd nearly forgotten there were other people in my life and other memories to consider. We traded stories while we took long, winding walks through the rice paddies, and it was almost like I was just getting to know her—this person I'd supposedly known my whole life. I wondered what else I had missed. What else didn't I know about all the people in my life who I loved but didn't talk to anymore?

Toward the end of the first week, one cup of coffee would condemn me to days of vomiting and pain. Bali belly. Sunny brought me plain rice and soup and we watched DVDs in our villa while I begged our stone Ganesha statue for mercy, but I could not peel myself away from the toilet. I could barely eat, but that didn't stop me from emptying my guts in bulk. I felt like I was exorcising demons.

Even after getting medication from the local clinic, I remained sick until the day we were slated to leave. I was in no mood to make a twentyish-hour trip in this condition. I didn't want to leave anyway. I hadn't seen everything I needed to. So I kissed Sunny goodbye before she left for the airport and I found myself a smaller place to stay, right next to a yoga studio called the Yoga Barn.

As Bali belly eased up, I took to meditating in the rice fields and practicing yoga daily. Although I'd tried meditating in the past, I never stuck with it because I couldn't ever keep my mind from wandering. Even though my mind still wandered, I was becoming better at bringing my attention back to the breath instead of following my thoughts wherever they took me—usually somewhere dark.

One teacher in Ubud taught me a clever trick. While meditating, I was to imagine myself sitting on the shores of a river. As I sat, boats passed by and I watched them come and go. The operative word here is *watched*. I didn't jump into the river and climb onto the boats. I didn't get carried away by them. These boats were my thoughts. I slowly learned to become aware of each thought as it entered my mind. Another recommendation, to make this awareness stronger, was to identify the thought. *Here's a fear thought. Here's a bored thought. Here's an angry thought.* When I became aware of the thought, I was less likely to attach myself to it and then I could return to my breath and a still mind, until the next thought came down the river.

My favorite yoga class was hatha-infused with tantric principles run by a tiny woman named Uma. At first, I had no idea what hatha meant; I had trouble distinguishing one yoga class from the next despite the variety of different "types" listed on studio schedules. Vinyasa seemed to involve more sun salutations. Anusara had the invocation. Restorative used lots of props. Kundalini exhausted me. And though I had practiced in New York and Hawaii, I didn't really consider myself a yogi because I had this idea swimming around in my head that yogis were enlightened people. They were healthy. They didn't sleep around or watch porn. They probably didn't even eat meat. I couldn't relate.

The first time I signed up for Uma's class, her devotees showed up first. These two pretty and serious young women sat with crossed legs at the front of the room. They didn't use yoga mats. They didn't chat with the students in class awaiting Uma. They sat in silence with their eyes closed until one of them emitted sound, either a buzz vibrating on her lips or a click cascading off her teeth. One would vigorously shake, while the other would gently tremble. One would laugh, the other would groan.

Some students in the class seemed unfazed. Maybe they knew what to expect. But the newbies stared at the girls and then searched each other's faces for an explanation. When Uma arrived, her wild hair framing her petite yet strong body, it was impossible not to feel the effects of her energy. There was a power to her presence that made it clear she was a master. Maybe it manifested in the way she carried herself into the room, sure of herself, awake.

"The aim of this class is to remove obstacles," she said, sitting down before us in lotus position. "You'll notice that those who are open and unlimited will express the natural flow of their energy through sound and movement. Do not fear these tendencies. To do so would mean fearing your own nature."

She took us through traditional salutations and I listened and watched as she and her devotees buzzed and clicked and convulsed. Some of the students in class went along with it, too. At one point, after a series of chants, Uma dropped to her stomach and burst into hysterical laughter. Nobody interrupted her. Nobody got up to leave. We just waited until she finished laughing, and then she sighed and stood up again. "You know what your greatest fear is?" she asked us.

One person shot back, "Death!"

"No," she said. "Not death. Your greatest fear is being exposed."

I made a habit out of attending Uma's class, determined to remove my obstacles and get comfortable with being exposed, no matter how terrifying that idea seemed. I was good at exposing sides of myself depending on whose bed I was in or how many drinks I'd had, but in everyday places and in everyday situations, how terrifying it was to simply be myself. I didn't even know who I was anymore.

Each class was similar in that Uma's devotees showed up first, strange sounds and movements sprung up from all directions of the room and she encouraged us, by example, to be our most authentic selves. Once, after one of her laughing fits, she declared in her booming voice, "In the West, to behave like this might land you in an institution. But in India, you're revered as a guru."

After each class I'd find myself in a different headspace than before. I was accustomed to the fleeting calmness that often occurred post-yoga and post-meditation. This was something else. Something much more powerful and full of possibility. I believed my Western mind was becoming, well, Eastern, in that what I had thought was Uma's madness in that very first class was now something natural. Something I wanted to possess.

Besides yoga, the Yoga Barn was also a source of healing sessions and Ayurvedic consultations at their rejuvenation center, Kush. I made an appointment with Uma for a consultation alluringly called "Know Thyself—Heal Thyself."

Though I was intrigued by Uma's prowess, I was still somewhat intimidated. I scheduled the consultation days in advance so that I could prepare myself for one-on-one time with her. I even scoured the internet for any information I could find that might make her more human in my eyes, less godly and superior.

In a 2010 interview with *The Jakarta Post*, I learned about Uma's extraordinary childhood in Kenya and about her retreat into the Balinese jungle, where she lived for seven years practicing yoga, consuming scorpion blood and drinking herbal aphrodisiacs.

"The most extraordinary miracle of all," she said, "is the profound genius of the human being in its capacity to grow."

◆

"I want to grow."

This is what I said when my one-on-one session with Uma finally came and I sat before her.

I had expected to feel intimidated by her, fearing that I might stumble over my words, try to impress her, and make myself appear foolish and weak in her presence. But it took just one smile from her and I let my guard down. She was warm now—still mighty as ever—but accessible, kind.

"OK, I'm going to ask you to think back," she said, pouring me a cup of ginger tea.

"How far back?" I asked, growing a bit wary.

"Before you started to change yourself for other people. Think back to your early youth. What were you like? What mattered to you?"

I thought back. Back before the boyfriends. Back before the porn. Back before the voice in my head started telling me I needed something outside of myself to feel happy. To feel satisfied. To feel anything at all. I talked about my curiosity. How badly I wanted to see the world. My hunger for adventure. My writing. I laughed because I suddenly remembered an old habit of talking to the mirror as a child. When I told Uma about that, she didn't laugh.

"This is a very advanced practice," she said. "Do you still do that?"

I thought about myself in various bathrooms around the world. Searching my body for imperfections. Masturbating with the water running so nobody would hear. I did more thinking than talking aloud and it was hardly positive thinking. "It's not the same," I told her. "I criticize myself much more."

She nodded. "I understand." Then she leaned forward in her

seat. "What is the thing, besides growth, that you're really looking for? Try to be specific."

I thought for a moment. It was difficult to pinpoint one single thing that I wanted. I felt overwhelmed by changing desires all the time. But I knew I wanted what Uma had. Her vitality, her confidence, her power. "I guess I want to find my power," I said.

I paused, leaving room for her to give me some priceless advice, some secret to the way she was.

Then she said, "You don't need to find anything, Erica. You need only to remember what you already have."

In efforts to expose myself, as scary as it seemed, I opened up to her about what had been going on with me.

"I never feel satisfied," I told her. "I jump from one relationship to the next, but I never feel worthy. The only pleasure I have is what my body can give me, but the pleasure never lasts. I feel empty and terrible about myself."

Her answer was simple. Go back, retrace, remember.

She sent me on my way with a prescription of books and yoga and self-care practices. And, last, an embrace that made my whole body vibrate with a new kind of energy. I wondered, was I feeling her energy or my own?

◆

I continued attending Uma's classes, but that wasn't all. It makes complete sense why Elizabeth Gilbert chose Ubud as her destination in Bali while she was on her mission to find herself. Ubud is full of opportunities for self-growth and learning and I took on the mentality I had in New York where I would try everything in my effort to live differently. What had changed was that now I wasn't trying to keep some man in my life. I was trying to reclaim a version of myself that was as powerful, centered, and aware as Uma.

I tried yoga nidra, or yoga sleep, with a woman who claimed to have cured her heart condition through deep meditation. I let a Balian, a traditional Balinese medicine man, rub toothpaste all over my belly and hit me in the head with a stick to promote my body's natural healing process. Through Reiki, a bearded man from San Francisco encouraged my energy to flow with vigor. Another bearded man, from San Diego, who was deep in silent practice, hugged me for nearly an hour to help me rediscover compassion.

Meeting people and connecting also became more appealing. Ubud was full of travelers, and everyone seemed to be on their own spiritual journey. I rode motorbikes with Mae from LA and chatted about love with Dina from Russia. Ethan was a flautist who divided his time between Ubud, Koh Phangan, and Goa, all places I would see one day, and be reminded of his playfulness. Lily had an alarm set in the daytime for every hour on the hour. When it rang, she jumped for joy and announced something for which she was grateful.

I also picked up the book *The Power Is Within You* by Louise L. Hay, which reiterated the importance of mirror work. She recommends greeting ourselves each morning with kind, encouraging messages. If something bad happened during the day, or we made some sort of mistake, she suggests running over to the mirror and reassuring ourselves, "All is OK. I love you anyway."

The first session of mirror work felt awkward. I wasn't sure I could be this person—this sane, calm, peaceful person who put herself first. But I was willing to at least give it a try without realizing how powerful this intention was. Nobody was watching me in my tiny Balinese bathroom, but I felt uncomfortable peering into my eyes so long and speaking aloud. It was almost as if my own reflection was some strange, distant girl I did not know. The first thing I said was, "I'm sorry." It wasn't long before the tears came. "I love you anyway," I said.

Like Hay suggested, I made a list of all the qualities I wanted to find in a relationship. I wanted someone on their own spiritual path, a yogi, a traveler, an artist, someone who was constantly reading and learning, someone honest, someone who was attentive and compassionate, someone I could trust to stick by me and hold me up when I fell and someone who would allow themselves to be held. Why didn't I deserve this?

◆

I remember everything about the first time I saw River in Uma's Sunday morning hatha class. His hair messy and damp from sweat. His eyes green and clear like shallow seawater. That familiar tug of interest radiating throughout my body and that voice inside my head, saying, *You're not ready. Not yet.*

I hadn't been romantically interested in anybody in Bali thus far. I hadn't even been that interested in porn, which was convenient, since the internet in Southeast Asia could be pretty spotty. All of my other self-serving efforts had taken precedence so that when the itch to watch porn sprang forward, I was more likely to divert my attention away from it, rather than give into it. This diverting action felt like an extension of my meditation practice.

And what relief there was in having a mind free from the searching, the scrolling, the coming, the hiding, and the emptiness that I always felt after I climaxed. I slept better. I was curious about the people around me. I was curious about myself and excited about all the things I wanted to see and do and write about.

I tried to divert my attention away from this attractive man in class, but that was proving to be more difficult, even with Uma standing there laughing, even with all the sun salutations and the sweating.

After one particular class, I rolled my mat up quickly, gathered my things, and headed to a nearby café, where I sat down with my Hay book and ordered a chai latte. A few moments later, there he was. I gulped.

He sat down at a nearby table and looked over the menu for a bit, before he turned his attention to me, sitting there quietly, trying not to stare at him.

"Have you ever had anything from the raw menu?" he asked.

"No, I haven't," I said. "Sorry."

That's when he got up and came to my table. "Do you mind?"

River was a jazz musician from Australia currently living in China. His parents were hippies from Nimbin, Australia's version of Woodstock, where they fought for rainforests and lived on a commune. His mother left him when he was a baby to follow the Indian mystic Osho, whom I didn't know much about, and so he was raised primarily by his father, a difficult man with a hearty appetite for weed and women. He talked about his time in New York, his travels to Thailand, how he was now training to be a yoga teacher. Then he asked about me. What book was I reading? What was I doing in Bali? Where had I been?

I felt like the whole world had quieted down to hear my answers. I wanted to speak my truth, to have an effortless connection with him like I'd had with so many of the other people I'd met in Bali thus far. I was ready now. I could be me.

But I felt my face grow hot and my voice quaver when I heard myself say, "I guess I'm sort of on a mission."

"What kind?" he asked, seeming genuinely interested.

The voice in my head that usually spoke up when I was uncomfortable told me to escape. To get the hell out of there because

I suddenly saw what it would all become. Our bodies naked in bed, the hollowness thereafter. He'd either break my heart or I'd break his. He'd lie to me. I'd use him.

"You know what?" I said, shooting up from my seat. "I just forgot I have somewhere to be. It was nice meeting you." I gathered my things and practically ran out of the café and away from him. I wasn't ready. No fucking way.

As if I'd learned nothing from my sessions with Uma or my meditation practice or my intense study of the Hay book, I followed my fear all the way to my bed, flipped open my laptop, and escaped. I started with pictures, just girls in bathing suits, their nipples covered. Then I took it a step further. Bare tits bouncing in short clips, girls rubbing oil all over their bodies. I was able to orgasm. When I regained my breath and the fear returned, I went for harder clips. Lesbians sharing a double dildo, their mouths hungrily lapping up each other's juices. Then a man and a woman fucking, tremendous grunting and groaning, an impressive eruption on her tits. I came again. I lay there, ashamed of myself for being back here, alone and afraid, instead of finding out what might have happened out there in the world with someone I found interesting. What if I was never ready?

The anxiety I felt thinking about my active compliance in my own isolation pushed me to a clip of two hot Latinas playing a faceless guy's cock like a harmonica. Suddenly I was the girl on the shore of that river I'd imagined in meditation. I watched a boat come by with a skinny blond college girl spread-eagle on its main deck getting fucked by a whole fraternity. And then another boat where a girl on a leash was held facedown by a man's boot while another man fucked her from behind. Each time I came, I returned to my breath, jagged and frantic. I found myself identifying the cacophony of my thoughts—fear thought, shame thought, guilt thought, hate thought, pity thought, hopeless thought. But the last time I came, it was so hard that I felt dizzy and sick. I slammed the laptop shut and slid it under my bed.

I got up, weak and quivering, and wobbled over to the bathroom, where I cleaned myself up with tissue and reluctantly stared at the mirror. I wanted to apologize to my tired reflection, but *Sorry* felt like too little. Instead, I said, "I'm out of control." I felt powerless. I hadn't yet been to a twelve-step meeting for sex, but I was already becoming acquainted with the very first step.

I carried my exhausted body over to the nearest spa and had a scalp massage with eucalyptus to ease my weary mind. Then I had lunch at a café that overlooked a rice field—a tomato and mozzarella salad with basil and olive oil. Hours had passed since I'd seen River, but I couldn't get him off my mind. What was the big deal? I seemed to be fixated on him the way I'd fixated on men in the past, but there was something different here. Two versions of myself arguing in my head about what this fixation was really about. Not whether he'd fuck me and whether I'd hate myself because of *how* he fucked me or *how often* he fucked me. No, this was all about curiosity. About him, of course, but also curiosity about myself.

How could I maintain the positivity I'd started building when faced with sexual attraction? How could I keep nourishing this calm, centered, kinder, and more aware person I'd only caught glimpses of in the past while opening up to another person who had the power to send me crashing down into all my old habits? Then the stronger voice in my head reminded me that he didn't actually have this power. I didn't have to give that to him.

I gobbled up my salad and ordered a sandwich too. I was ravenous. And I was slightly embarrassed to be having this battle in my head, feeling like I was sinking into neurosis because of some brief interaction with a stranger. I felt naive, like a child, needy for attachment. But then I had a hippie thought, very appropriate for a place like Ubud—if it was in the universe's plan for something to actually happen with River, then the universe would plan to send him my way again. With that thought, I surrendered and found some peace for the remainder of my lunch.

I finished my sandwich, paid, and exited the café. Once I was back on the uneven pavement lined with mala bead shops, juice bars, and yoga boutiques, there was River, mounting his motorbike.

Terrified, but excited, I ran over to him. He was heading back to the place where he was staying, about an hour's drive away, but he'd be back in a few days if I wanted to hang out.

"Do you have any plans?" he asked.

◆

Days later, we sipped kombucha together in the rice fields at a place called Sari Organik while we talked about our lives. Not just the lives that brought us together in this foreign place, but also the lives we were aiming to have. We both wanted to see the world more. To learn what we didn't yet know from people and places we hadn't yet encountered. We talked with enthusiasm, and I felt relaxed with him, awake and alive.

At some point he told me he was an addict, sober for two years. He'd dabbled in numerous drugs and drank too much, but the drug that finally drove him to seek help was actually not seen as a drug by many.

"It's kind of embarrassing," he said.

"Embarrassing how?"

"Well, for a long time, I didn't think you could be addicted to pot," he said, laughing. "But so much of my life's happiness was sucked away because of this habit I just couldn't kick. I'd talked myself out of seeking help for so long because I was convinced that what I was doing wasn't so bad. It wasn't like I was shooting heroin or anything."

It seemed to me that porn and masturbation were the pot of sex addiction. And sex addiction was probably the pot of all addictions. After all, you can't die from a whole day in bed with a joint or streaming porn clips. But life slips through your wet and achy fingers anyway.

As we talked, I noticed how romantic it all was. Our bodies close, talking about real things. The sun setting over the rice paddies, palm trees swaying in the distance, farmers working on their land, butterflies and the scent of jasmine filling the air. One giant black butterfly wouldn't leave me alone. It flapped around my face and drink until bravely settling on my hand.

"How cool," he said, gently touching the butterfly with his finger. "Do you know what black butterflies symbolize?"

"No," I said, shaking my hand a bit so the butterfly would fly away. I was not a fan of insects, even beautiful and harmless ones. The creature didn't flinch.

He laughed. "I'm not sure either. But I think it's something important."

Later that night I looked up the black butterfly online and learned that many cultures believe it is an omen of death. But most believe it symbolizes transition and rebirth encapsulated in its fluttering, delicate presence.

◆

Hours later, we lay naked in bed.

I was somehow able to overcome the fear and awkwardness that usually permeates a first lovemaking session so that it was enjoyable and tender. Afterward, facing each other with our limbs entangled, he said, "This might be a big thing to say, but I know I'm ready for this."

This. I wasn't sure what he meant. Awesome sex? Did he want to go again?

"Ready for what?"

"I'm ready to let love into my life. How about you?"

Everything inside of me wanted to scream, "Yes! Of course! I'm ready!" But I kissed him instead, and we fell asleep.

I awoke early the next morning in a panic. It was still dark outside but I needed him to leave so I could be alone. I gently tapped him on the arm. "River, wake up. I have to work early."

It was a lie, but I figured that like most men I'd slept with before, he'd appreciate the easy out regardless of what he said the night before in his postcoital daze. No obligation to cuddle me or buy me breakfast or spend the whole day making small talk. I wasn't that type of girl. I even pointed to my laptop on the desk to stress the urgency of my need for space. It was plugged in and fully charged, ready to distract me however I wanted it to.

Half asleep, he nodded and mumbled something, but he made no effort to get up and leave. I didn't tap him again. Instead, I slumped back onto my pillow and listened to him breathing, steady and full. His mind was definitely far away from me and my fear. I thought about nudging him harder until he woke up, sighing loudly or leaving a note on the bedside table like they do in movies. But I didn't move. I just listened to his breathing. Slowly, light filled the room, illuminating our scattered clothes across the floor and our bodies in a tight embrace. Eventually, I fell back to sleep.

Throughout the next few days, my panic subsided enough so that we could enjoy each other. We rode his motorbike all over Bali, my hands gripped around his waist, crossing bridges and jungly paths to arrive at secluded beaches with mighty waves. We drank coconuts and ate fresh fish and got to know each other more, pausing only to make out or, if we were alone in my room, make love. But the panic often returned in the early mornings when River was deep in sleep and I was deep in worry. It was difficult to pinpoint what exactly I was worried about. I was good about identifying my thoughts so far and this definitely felt like fear, but fear over what? Fear he might hurt me? Fear I might hurt him? There was no sign pointing to something bad happening between us. He was open with his feelings and seemed to be everything I'd been searching for. He'd made his own list of the qualities he wanted in a partner—and I measured up.

◆

River told me work was calling him back to China just a week into our romance. I felt relief. This thing between us could remain petite and perfect, untainted by what usually happens with romance—disappointment, pain, boredom.

But then he said the unexpected.

"You should come to Shanghai."

Without giving myself too long to think about it, I agreed. "I *should* go. I will go." I pulled him close and kissed his mouth.

Inside, my heart thumped hard and my stomach ached, but I repeated in my head what I felt to be most true. *I should go despite how scared I am. I should go because I'm curious about him. I should go because I'm curious about who I could be with him.*

So I followed him.

I said good-bye to the free-spirited expats I sat next to in cafés and stretched next to on the yoga mat. I said good-bye to the statues of Ganesha, the temples with their gamelan players and Ubud's enchanting rice fields. And I took one more class with

Uma, basking in her powerful energy just one last time before I faced the outside world again. I was scared to leave, but I tried to convince myself this fear was good for me. I wanted to be brave and bold. I wanted to take chances.

What I didn't expect was that River in Shanghai was not River in Bali. And Erica in Shanghai wasn't Erica in Bali either. From the moment my taxi deposited me at his apartment, we both realized how big and scary it all was.

"No one has ever made a gesture like this for me," he said, as if it made him suspicious. "No one's ever traveled from another country just to be with me. Are you sure you want to be here?"

He seemed insecure and fidgety, definitely not as affectionate or warm as he'd been before.

This made me respond with my own insecurity. And while all of my fear was still there as it had been in Bali, it wasn't just in my head anymore. I was either reactionary and mean or distant and cold. I told him stories about past lovers, but not in a confessional way. I boasted. He did the same. He sighed heavily when I didn't take out my wallet to pay for things, but I didn't care. Our conversations led to dead ends and we ran out of things to do together quickly, so I felt I had nothing to reach for except what I'd always reached for to help me with the awkwardness. I initiated sex whenever I felt things getting weird. I was tireless with blow jobs, encouraging him to come on my face, begging him to slap me, to fuck me harder, to hurt me, to do whatever he wanted, playing the role of the perfect, pleasing porn girl.

He was into it, but only for so long. Eventually, it was obvious that he wanted me to leave, and it was obvious to me that I was tired of this dumb old role. I bought my ticket back to LA. He didn't protest.

◆

Back at my parents' house, I wasn't sure what I should do next or where I should go or who I should call. It was a familiar feeling—not knowing—but instead of the situation causing me distress as it always had in the past, I was amused with myself. I had been here so many times—through with some guy or some place and back at square one. I was like a hamster on a wheel or Sisyphus on his mountain, and I was tired of it.

I wasn't even back two weeks when I received an email from River apologizing for how things went down in Shanghai. He confessed to being scared and insecure and said that the whole experience had helped open his eyes to how unhappy he was in China. He'd decided to move—maybe go to Thailand or India or back to Bali, anywhere but where he was. I apologized too. I'd also been scared. It was such a relief to say the truth.

With safe distance between us, I revealed more. Days before, I'd been watching TV late at night and caught Steve McQueen's film *Shame* starring Michael Fassbender.

I watched his character, Brandon, jerk off in his work bathroom after flirting with a woman on a train. I watched him fail to get an erection with a woman he actually cared for because he didn't know how to bridge sex and human connection. I watched him get fellated by a man in a club, lose his shit when his sister accidentally walks in on him masturbating in the shower, and break down in tears when he realizes he has lost control.

"I think I'm a sex addict," I wrote to River, feeling exposed but brave behind the protection of my computer screen. Though I'd secretly believed this for some time now, I'd never actually confessed it to another person.

He wrote back, "That makes a lot of sense, actually," noting

my distance during sex, my lack of eye contact and my tendency
to pull away when things got too intimate. He confessed that my
sex drive had intimidated him in Shanghai and so had my stories
about other men. But hearing his assessment of me was too much,
so I did what was expected—I pulled away.

He wouldn't leave me alone though. He was full of apologies,
and I was full of confessions, and our email exchanges grew more
intense. He also had a ton of questions. What was I going to do
now? Where was I going to go? Would I like to meet up again?

I thought about who we were in Bali and how positive that
part of our story had been. But because everything had fallen apart
in Shanghai, the story had changed. And now that I was in LA,
the story was changing even more and becoming less tangible. I
couldn't decide if I'd built everything up too much in Bali, if he
was someone I could trust, or if I was ready after all.

I tried to ignore him, focusing instead on what I wanted to do—
how to make the most of where I was before deciding where to go
from there. I decided, fueled by my reluctant admission, to stop
masturbating, cold turkey. This seemed preposterous, because
even when I'd watched so little porn in Bali, I hadn't thought to
kick masturbation. After all, Hay writes in *The Power Is Within
You*, "The moment you are willing to change, it is remarkable how
the Universe begins to help you. It brings you what you need."

I really wanted to believe that.

◆

One of the things that helped me keep my hands out of my pants
and my browser history clean throughout the next couple of
months was attending my first ever SLAA meetings. Paranoid of
what they'd think, I told my parents I was working in cafés all day
and night; they didn't seem suspicious anyway.

The first meeting was held in a basement of a church in Silver Lake. There were multiple groups meeting at the same time when I arrived—Narcotics Anonymous in one room, Alcoholics Anonymous in another—so I stumbled awkwardly into a few of the wrong ones before I found my people. And right away, they felt like my people. Many of them restless, self-deprecating, distant. At least that's how I perceived them. There were mostly men at this meeting—only three women including me—and I tried to avoid all of their eyes, attempting to make myself invisible in the corner. I wasn't ready to admit that I was a sex addict to a group of strangers, and I had already prepared a speech beforehand in case anyone questioned me. "I'm just curious," I'd say. But nobody questioned me. They went through the twelve steps and twelve traditions I would come to know so well, and then one of them read a passage aloud. I listened and nodded, thinking, *Yes, that sounds like me. Yes, that could be me. Yes, that's definitely me.*

When the floor opened to shares, I focused on my hands on my lap, paranoid someone would call on me. I hated speaking aloud in groups, and I was in no way ready to speak here. But, again, nobody called on me. SLAA meetings weren't like other social circles or intimidating classrooms where I often felt inferior in what I had to offer. There was no pressure to offer anything. There was no pressure to do or be anything that I didn't want to be or I wasn't ready to be. So I listened, soaking up the confessions of others, their vulnerability and their humor and their desperation. And what surprised me most was the similarity of their shares. This similarity would remain throughout most of the other meetings I'd attend in other cities and countries over the years.

While women often talked about avoiding sex and relationships, men tended to talk about seeking sex and temporary relationships, but for the exact same reasons—fear of intimacy. Not every case was the same. Whether the women talked about how many years had passed since they last shared a bed with another warm body, or the men talked about how many prostitutes they slept with over the last year, it almost always came back to a feeling of isolation fueled by fear. And this fear was often fueled by a feeling of unworthiness. And this feeling of unworthiness could almost always be traced back to an early memory. We had all learned, at some point, to believe a lie about ourselves—that we were bad, or ugly, or broken, or unlovable, and now we were seriously questioning that lie. Now, we wanted to unlearn it.

When other addicts shared about porn addiction, my ears always perked up. Porn kept us from engaging with the world. Porn distorted our perception, not just of sex, but of everything. Something so simple, like standing in an elevator with other people, or brushing up against another body on the subway, or exchanging money with a supermarket clerk—anything really—could quickly be turned into a pornographic scene by our trained, overstimulated minds. We felt numb to touch and always craved more of it. We were impatient and disinterested with a situation unless it was leading to sex. We were never really satisfied with the act of sex—it could always be better—and when it was over, we quickly wanted to discard the person. Their use was diminished. *Our* use was diminished.

After a few weeks of no orgasms and regular meetings, where I continued to avoid sharing, I was hypersensitive and emotional. I found comfort in hearing other people's stories, feeling less isolated whenever something resonated with me, but I was slightly discouraged by the "powerless" theme that ran through every meeting. Although I felt powerless at the moment, my abstinence from orgasms being new and unfamiliar, I didn't want to believe that I'd *always* feel this way. I wanted to believe my cravings would subside one day and that I'd somehow be able to find moderation with my sexuality. But this didn't seem likely in any of the meetings, as comforting as they were for me. It didn't matter if an addict had been attending meetings for two months or two years or longer, they still had to proclaim their powerlessness over sex and love addiction when reciting the twelve steps. And they still had to devote themselves to some external force, whether it was God or some other higher power.

Though I wasn't masturbating, I couldn't keep from fantasizing about sex, ruminating over how things went with River and all the sex we'd had in Shanghai, and I still wasn't sure what to do about him as we continued to exchange emails and chat online. Like my use of porn, I felt attached to the screen, but also safely distant. I could shut the laptop and walk away when I wanted. It was easier this way, but also not entirely fulfilling. This was not real intimacy, and I knew that. I was playing it safe by not answering his questions about whether I'd meet up with him again, somewhere in the world, choosing instead to focus on my day-to-day avoidance of sexual pleasure and burying myself in work and distraction.

Almost every interaction in my life, around this time, felt distant, like a halfway effort. I went to the screen, not just for brief interactions with River, but for everything. I still worked online, writing copy for the agency I worked for in New York, only communicating with my coworkers through email, and with friends through social media platforms like Facebook and Instagram. Online, I could be whoever I wanted to be, project a happy and interesting version of my life, but in reality, loneliness persisted.

I couldn't distract myself from my emotions, though. I was in the midst of my second month of complete abstinence when two

things happened: my grandma died suddenly of a heart attack and
I met a guy at Starbucks named Chris.

My mom took her mother's death extremely hard. She'd had a
complex relationship with her and too much was left unsaid and
unresolved in the end. I took her death hard too, but it was even
more difficult to figure out how best to support my mom, who
was inconsolable. I retreated from the house as much as possible,
working at the nearby Starbucks and attending even more SLAA
meetings just to get away from all of the heightened emotions I felt
ill equipped to manage.

I didn't seek Chris out. There were no empty tables that day
and I needed to plug in my laptop and work. But it seemed to
be in my DNA to gravitate toward the most attractive man wherever I was. Hours later, we were in my car driving to a nearby bar,
him flattering me the way men do when they've been successful
too many times flattering women all the way to bed. We didn't
sleep together that day though. Or any other day over the next few
weeks where we drank together and I let him pull me close, whispering in my ear all the things he'd like to do to me if only I'd let
him. But I didn't let him because I was adamant about this newfound commitment of avoiding sexual pleasure. To ensure chas-
tity without a medieval belt, I emailed River and told him I'd like
to meet up with him a few days after Christmas, a whole month
away. We decided on Thailand.

I also told him about how well I'd been doing managing my
sex addiction, attending SLAA meetings and avoiding other men,
hoping this made me more appealing in his eyes, a clean and worthy candidate of his love. We made an oath to each other not to
sleep with anyone else like two high school kids sliding purity
rings on each other's fingers.

Then I shut my computer and didn't talk to him for weeks,

continuing to go out with Chris just to see if I could uphold my oath as much as I wanted to break it. During one of these weeks, at one of my SLAA meetings, an attractive woman with bleached-blond hair and a low-cut tank shared her salacious weekend with the group. She'd answered yet another ad on Craigslist and had sex with yet another group of strangers and she was sure she had contracted yet another STD. She didn't seem ashamed or regretful of what had transpired. Instead, she seemed resigned to her impulses. Like maybe the act of confessing would one day be the catalyst to make her finally change, even if her body wasn't there yet.

Few women at the meetings had shared details about their promiscuity and I found her story unsettling. I couldn't help but compare myself to her, feeling too many things at once. Envious of her exciting weekend. Intimidated by her attractiveness. Confused by her hunger.

Dumbfounded, I went home and masturbated, first imagining the woman at her orgy, and then imagining myself as the woman. I came so hard I thought my heart might explode. Afterward, I crawled under the covers and cried. I hadn't decided how long I was going to keep from having an orgasm, but this didn't feel like enough time. And with River waiting in the wings and Chris blowing up my phone, I already knew what came next. The incessant reach for more and more and more with the knowledge that I'd never change no matter how hard I tried. I wanted, desperately, to remain pure and as perfect as possible for River, even though we weren't talking that much. Even talking to him seemed dangerous. What if I ruined things before we had our second shot?

To ensure I kept my oath of not sleeping with anyone, I stopped seeing Chris. I also stopped attending the SLAA meetings because I didn't want to be triggered again by another person like the bleached-blond woman. More than that, I didn't want to keep telling myself, even if it felt true, that I was an addict. I was scared that the admission would become a justification to act out—isn't that what addicts do? I counted down the days until I saw River again. The only thing left to do in LA was do nothing at all.

nine

THE GIRL INSIDE

Walking around Bangkok, nearly everywhere you look, you'll find "massage parlors" where women sit behind glass as if in a fish bowl, waiting for their next client to choose them. They stand on streets holding signs over their heads: *Free Blow Job with Drink!* They launch Ping-Pong balls out of their orifices for iPhone cameras in dingy, darkened bars. They follow old men back to their hotel rooms. They follow young men too.

Prostitution has been illegal in Thailand since 1960, but a tourist wouldn't know this.[15] Some $16 million of foreign soldiers' money went toward Thai prostitution during the Vietnam War, igniting a tourist industry with a seedy reputation the country hasn't been able to shake.

I'd heard about Thailand's prostitution scene before visiting,

---

15 A black-market study by Havocscope in 2015 found that the illegal practice is estimated to be worth $6.4 billion a year in revenue and is a large part of the country's GDP.

but I had no idea how prevalent it really was. And with this new idea that I might be a sex addict flying around in my head, it seems absurd now that I would agree to meet there at that delicate moment in time. Luckily, River had arranged for us to spend just one tantalizing week in Bangkok, which I naively thought was the only place we'd see prostitutes, before flying to the island of Koh Phangan for a tantra festival based on Osho's teachings. This sounded more like the kind of thing I should be doing.

But I'd be lying if I didn't admit to my curiosity, which quickly became my craving, for the so-called massage parlors and girl bars and scantily clad women of Bangkok's street corners. While I never saw Western women like myself leading one of these women back to their hotel rooms or inquiring the prices of the shadiest massage parlors, I wondered—would the women serve me if I approached? Or would they laugh at me?

I couldn't ask River about any of this, of course. When he picked me up from Bangkok's Suvarnabhumi Airport and held me tight in his arms, I felt the same warmth I'd felt in Bali that first romantic week.

"It's so good to see you again," he said. Then he pulled away to look me in the eyes and he kissed me. He was softer now, relaxed. "I'm happy we're giving this another shot."

"Me too," I said. I was still nervous but also relieved. It felt right to be there with him. I was excited about what might happen between us and even more excited to be in a new city again. And I was proud of myself for having kept my oath and not slept with anyone, as tempted as I'd been at times.

We took a taxi to our hotel, making out in the backseat most of the time. When I came up for air, I was overwhelmed by the madness of the streets. Not just the girls in their miniskirts and spiky heels, but the endless vendors selling their goods: bootleg

DVDs and quirky T-shirts, any pharmaceutical you could think of, sex toys, incense, sunglasses, sarongs. All that to look at, plus the intense smells of fried fish, tropical fruits, and rich curries. And, of course, the cacophony of car horns, loud music playing, motorbikes flying past—so much stimuli that I was glad to finally be locked away from it in our underpriced hotel room.

We stayed in bed for what seemed like days, eating chicken satay on sticks and drinking from fresh coconuts between countless lovemaking sessions. He talked as he had in Bali, telling me how ready he was for love. I told him I was ready too, and I wanted to believe it. More than that, I wanted to be completely comfortable with him, to believe that he was into me as much as I was into him. I wanted to be confident and secure in my own skin, a strong and powerful woman who knew her worth, but the more he talked, the more fascinating he became and the more I feared he'd bolt if he knew what was underneath the pretty smile he loved to compliment and the calm and pleasant demeanor I showed him.

He was interested in so many different cultures and told vivid stories. He was talented and spiritual and funny and attractive, and though he'd seemed grumpy and annoyed with me in Shanghai, I couldn't pinpoint any serious flaws yet, and without those flaws I couldn't help but feel inferior. What if he figured me out?

Back home, when I had confessed to him through email that I might be a sex addict and he didn't seem surprised, I was quick to pull away and spare him the details. If I didn't reveal too much, then he could imagine the most minor offenses. And while I ran the risk of him imagining worse things than I'd ever done, without any confirmation on my part, he couldn't know for sure. If I could prove to him how whole and sane and polite I was, maybe he'd forget I'd made that confession to him in the first place.

Sex with him was tender and fulfilling. We couldn't get enough of each other. I felt like I had when we were back in Bali and I was convinced that the awkwardness of Shanghai had been a glitch in our story. When we weren't in the hotel room naked, we were out getting our feet rubbed and feasting like kings for a few bucks. At one point, he left me alone so he could go to a twelve-step meeting, and I wandered around the streets, trying to pay attention to the shops and street vendors. But I was more interested in what they were selling in the types of places that advertised: *Massage by Model* or *Soapy Massage*.

I found myself climbing the steps of one of these places near Nana Plaza, one of Bangkok's most notorious red-light districts, moving quickly, practically running so I wouldn't change my mind. "I'll just have a look inside," I told myself. It was day, but the inside of the building was dark, illuminated only by sultry red bulbs. About twenty girls with identical red dresses and clear, plastic heels sat behind a pane of glass, their mouths shut, waiting.

"Can I help you?" An older Thai woman dressed in black approached me. She handed me a menu, which had various stages of sex at shockingly low payment—hand job being the cheapest service, which was depicted with a cartoon drawing of a hand and a penis, then hand job with a topless girl, hand job with a fully naked girl, blow job, and sex. All depicted in cartoons, which seemed comical.

My heart racing, I studied the menu and then glanced over at the girls, then down again.

"They can't see you," the woman assured me. "Take a closer look."

I walked over to the glass and saw that I wanted them all. But despite what the woman had said, I felt like they were looking right at me. Blank stares instead of confusion or disgust, which I appreciated, but not openness or kindness either. What did I expect? Some girl to jump up and beg me to choose her? A new BFF with benefits? My desperation sickened me.

Feeling too self-conscious, I handed the menu back to the woman and got out of the place as quickly as I'd entered. Bangkok was too dangerous for me, I decided. I needed to leave before I did something I could never take back.

◆

A month later, River and I were in a hotel room in Koh Samui fucking in front of my open laptop, our eyes glued to a clip of two big-titted Latinas taking turns sucking off one lucky guy. Sometimes they sucked at the same time—one working the head, the other the balls—and I could tell that excited him the most.

"They're like puppies going for the teat," he said.

He was right. That's exactly what they looked like. And thinking of them like animals was the last little push I needed to have an orgasm. After I had rubbed myself to satisfaction and let out a telling sigh, he came too and then collapsed next to me on the bed. I closed the laptop shut on the nightstand.

We hadn't lasted long at the tantra festival in Koh Phangan— just three days instead of the full week we paid for. It was enough time to practice eye gazing with total strangers, grunt like gorillas in front of a room full of people to get in touch with our animalistic sides, and crawl around like babies, babbling senseless sounds to engage with our childhoods. We'd turned our bodies into pretzels in yoga, meditated for hours, chanted sacred mantras, massaged each other, and danced together. But every time River and I looked at each other, we'd laugh. We weren't feeling it. I was used to the hippie stuff in Bali and had expected the tantra festival to be more of that, but this just felt like too much. I respected the enthusiasm of the other participants—they seemed moved by everything—but I couldn't help but feel like I was faking it. River felt the same way.

So we decided to go to the neighboring island of Koh Samui, renting a bungalow for just $300 a month near Lamai Beach. One of the largest of Thailand's islands, Koh Samui is known for its palm-lined beaches and mountainous rainforest, but it's also home to a racy nightlife scene with the same kind of massage parlors and girl bars you might find in Bangkok. We lived near a street we came to call "Hooker Street." It was the type of place where women advertised themselves all day and night in miniskirts and midriff tops, bright pink Hula-Hoops orbiting their tanned bare waists.

River didn't know how tempted I'd been by all the girl bars and massage parlors in Bangkok. I hadn't told him. As far as he was concerned, my biggest problems had been with porn and casual sex in my twenties, but I told him SLAA had worked wonders for me. I was happier now. I had learned self-control.

When I wasn't working, I spent a lot of time walking up and down that street, trying not to stare at the women or feel jealous when they called out to the men who walked past, never calling out to me. I was not their target customer. River spent much of his time at the nearby Muay Thai gym, perfecting his kicks and elbow jabs while small but impressively strong and sculpted Thai men held pads for him.

Back in bed with him, I'd finally found satisfaction with the help of his body, my fingers, the Latina porn stars, and the memories of all the Thai girls who paid no attention to me earlier in the day.

"What's your favorite porn scene?" he suddenly asked.

It was an unexpected question, and I had no desire to answer it. I thought we were going to nap or cuddle for a while until we were ready to go again.

"Why do you ask?" I reached for the sheet, damp with sweat, and yanked it up to cover my breasts.

"I don't know," he said. "Curiosity?" He turned over on his side and propped his head up on his left hand. His green eyes were wide with wonder.

The possibilities of what I could say ran through my head. I thought it best to describe something plain, something like a busty blonde getting banged by her personal trainer, or two hot teens bent over their math teacher's desk. These were the most harmless answers I could think of. Racy, but not demented. Hot, but not disgusting.

But they were lies. Maybe it was better to not say anything at all.

"Seems like a weird question," I said. I tucked the sheet into my armpits and scooted my body a little to the left so we were no longer touching. The tone of my voice was now defensive.

"It's just that I usually pick the porn," he explained. "Do you like what I choose?"

"Yeah, sure." I looked up at the ceiling. "They're fine."

"Are you sure?"

I suddenly understood what was happening. He was feeling guilty about getting off to porn while having sex with me and he was trying to reconnect. Even more, he was trying to get to know me on some deeper level. And what could be deeper than knowing a person's favorite porn scene? It's much more significant than a person's favorite category, full of endless options of soon-to-be-unexciting material. But a person's favorite porn scene? Porn is meant to be consumed and then discarded. There's no need to keep watching the same scene over and over when there's so much available all the time. With that much novelty at your disposal, why would anyone return to any one clip enough times to consider it a favorite? How could one scene maintain its appeal?

Yet, with all the porn I'd watched over the years and all the categories I'd gotten bored with, I *did* have a favorite scene. A scene so troubling and stomach-turning that the idea of telling him seemed like the most dangerous thing I could do. If he knew what really turned me on, he'd know that it must have taken quite a pitiful journey to get there. And if he knew how much porn I really watched, he'd know just how pathetic I really was. And if I was that pathetic, something must be wrong with me. Maybe he'd start asking about everything else.

As much as I wanted to pull the covers completely over my head and be swallowed up by the bed or teleported to some other place, there was a part of me that couldn't ignore how important this moment was. Too many of my past relationships, romantic or otherwise, were doomed by my inability to tell the whole truth, to fully be myself. Now I had the opportunity to go there, and to say to a person, *This is who I am. Do you accept me?*

"Well, there's this one gang bang," I started, looking over at his face to see a reaction of surprise and interest register at once.

"Go on."

I took a deep breath and proceeded to tell him, first slowly, then progressively faster about the scene. I could hardly hold back the rush of descriptors that fumbled from my mouth: two women, fifty men, a warehouse, a harness, a hair dryer and a taxicab. All put together in the most unexpected and enticing spectacle of degradation I've ever seen.

I watched his expression morph from one of interest to revulsion until I finally finished speaking.

For a long moment, there was silence between us, but there was also a sense of relief on my part. I had revealed something so dark, so upsetting, so impacted in shame, and he hadn't pulled away. He was still there beside me, propped up on his left hand, naked and vulnerable, and so was I. He saw me and I saw him, and we were in new territory.

But then he said, "I kind of wish I hadn't asked." It was all I needed to hear to send me into tears. Not just tiny, embarrassed sobs, but humiliated wails—a tantrum. Confused, he pulled me close to him, laughing nervously at my abrupt shift in disposition. I tried to pull the sheet over me, but he pulled it back down and covered my face with apologetic kisses. He couldn't possibly understand why I was crying, that what I'd just revealed to him was something I'd never shared with anyone.

"What's going on? Baby, what's wrong?"

And so I told him. How long I'd been watching porn like this. How I couldn't get turned on unless I was turned off. How I needed the women to be mistreated and misused—guzzling gallons of cum, slapped, thrown around, laughed at, walked around on leashes, ridiculed, dragged by their hair and tossed into the Dumpster. Anything that announced to the world that they were worthless and deserved to be humiliated. Because I felt worthless. I deserved to be humiliated. Porn was a mirror for how I felt about myself, a sexual being who couldn't stop rubbing herself numb, who let guys fuck her into oblivion, who hungered after the Thai girls on the street and the men who purchased them, who hungered after anything that might quiet her mind for a few moments and satiate the itch that never seemed to go away.

"But you're not worthless," he assured me. "Why would you ever think that?"

That was the question, wasn't it? Where had I learned the lie that I'd been telling myself for so long that I could no longer see an alternative?

◆

We decided to stop watching porn while we made love. Even calling it "making love" seemed a wild shift in a new direction. To my surprise, vaginal orgasms were no longer impossible, and I didn't have to touch myself or daydream to get there. Sensations felt brand-new, like when I used to get high on pot before having sex. I got high on our connection now, which grew stronger with every confession we made to each other, every honest word we uttered.

I also started to cut down the amount of porn I watched when River wasn't with me, taking my work to cafés so I wouldn't be tempted, practicing yoga and sometimes joining him at the Muay Thai gym, where I sweated out my frustrations through right hooks, uppercuts, and diagonal knees. There was a new kind of gratification in using my body this way. It was almost like sex—an outlet for release—but after a Muay Thai session I didn't feel empty. I felt energized. I didn't want to crawl into a hole and die. I wanted to pound my feet on the pavement like I'd pounded my fists against the pads, walking with purpose, announcing my presence, feeling the strong support of the earth beneath my weight.

I found myself easing up around him, feeling more secure and safe and having so much fun I thought we could live in Koh Samui forever, paying pennies for day-to-day luxury, my body getting stronger by the minute, my head clearer than it had ever been. I was happy.

Then he told me about the girl.

We were eating Indian *thali* plates, a refreshing diversion from the green curry and fish cakes and papaya salad we usually shared. I was talking about how long it had been since we last watched porn. That got me talking about the break I'd taken from it in LA when we were separated. That led to me mentioning the SLAA meetings and boasting about how I'd stayed pure for him.

"No sex for three months," I said. It was the longest I'd ever gone since I lost my virginity at seventeen. It was completely out of character and a big deal for me.

I'd told him this before—several times—but I still hadn't gotten the reaction or recognition I needed. I needed him to understand what this meant. That I liked him so much, I'd make a promise like that and keep it. After all that I'd confessed to him recently, he should know what a sacrifice that was. I was a girl who really liked sex. Who didn't just like sex but depended on it. And even though I hoped he knew how much I liked him, I considered this sacrifice of mine the ultimate confirmation, the grandest of gestures, just in case he didn't trust me yet.

A look came over his face. I knew shame when I saw it. I knew it intimately, like an extra limb.

"I should tell you something," he said.

I braced myself.

"There was a girl just before we met up."

I felt like someone had punched me in the gut. "Tell me everything," I said, against my better judgment.

He resisted, but I demanded. Her name. Where she was from. What she looked like. What they did. I hated knowing the details, but somehow I needed them. And each word he reluctantly shared only pieced together terrible images in my head that I knew would stay there for a long time. I got up from the table, no longer hungry, and he got up too, digging in his pocket for money to leave on the table. His eyes brimmed with tears and his breathing went jagged as he tried to explain to the back of my body how sorry he was.

Out on the street, I waved for a motorbike taxi, my own eyes filling with tears, my head heavy, my heart heavier. River ran out after me, excuses falling from his lips—his lips that had made a promise he couldn't keep, that had been on me and also on her. I wanted him to die. I wanted her to die.

I wanted to die. What a naive, pathetic fool to think he was an honest man. To think he was a good man. Of course he wasn't a good man. Good men were not for me.

"We weren't talking that much," he tried to explain as I climbed onto the back of a motorbike. "I got scared. I didn't think this was real! Or that I could trust you." I gave our address to the taxi driver and sped away without looking back.

When I returned to the bungalow, I went straight to the laptop. But instead of reaching for porn, I reached for something more painful—pictures of her. I searched for her name on Facebook, and I found some young and beautiful thing that I was sure he liked more than me. Now I had a face and body to put together with the painful details he'd provided, painting an even clearer picture of what they'd done together.

I took these images to the bed and masturbated myself into a stupor of humiliation and self-pity. I thought about the adrenaline coursing through his body as he made one bad decision after the next. The gratification of handing himself over to his lust. The secret weighing on him when we met up and I'd first boasted to him about what a good girl I'd been.

When he made it back, I wasn't masturbating anymore. I was crying. He was crying too. He dropped to his knees on the side of the bed and begged me to forgive him. He was a terrible person, he admitted. He'd made a horrible mistake and he hated himself for it.

"I love you," he said over and over. "I don't want to lose you. Please tell me I haven't lost you."

There was a part of me that wanted to land an uppercut on his chin the way the Muay Thai trainers had instructed me. To run away to a new place, justified by his dishonesty and my idea of what a jilted woman should do if ever in this position.

Another part of me, a less familiar part, wanted to console him, to pull him close and tell him that I understood. To forgive the unforgiveable. It was true we'd only had that one romantic week in Bali and that completely unromantic week in Shanghai. We were practically strangers during those three months apart.

But how could I forgive someone when I had never truly forgiven myself for all the lies I'd ever told, all the boundaries I'd consciously crossed, and all the people I'd hurt along the way, including myself?

◆

I got drunk nearly every day for two weeks after he told me, having belligerent arguments with him that I remember only in fragments. I picked up sleeping pills from the nearby pharmacy, hung out among boisterous tourists in girl bars, and tried desperately to shut off my mind. We fucked too, but I hardly remember that either. I know I must have also worked during the day, but I can't imagine that I produced anything satisfactory. I'm still surprised I didn't lose my job.

When I escaped his presence and told him not to follow me, I always ended up on Hooker Street. I worked up the courage to enter those alluring massage parlors, ignoring the confused looks of the half-dressed women who always called out to the men. But to my disappointment, they only ever massaged me. I was too shy to ask for more than that, sighing in dissatisfaction when they worked out my shoulder knots and never rubbed higher than my upper thighs.

"I want you to pick up a girl for me," I told River one Saturday, after I'd had a few margaritas.

"Um, OK," he said carefully, seeming concerned but not wanting to upset me. I think he would have done anything at that point to win back my favor. Even though we were fucking, we were fighting much more. My anger was palpable.

I didn't want to go back to Hooker Street because I didn't want to run into the woman we chose after we'd finished with her. So he drove us a little farther, to another street that looked just as scandalous.

He stopped in front of one of the massage parlors, where six or seven women sat out front, their dark skin glowing in the sunshine.

"Wait here," he said, leaving me straddling the motorbike, balancing the weight and power between my legs while he asked the price, a short conversation. The woman he chose spoke little English, so he negotiated with her boss, a fortyish woman in jean shorts and a tank top, her cleavage prominent. She said, through a thick accent: *You take her.*

We did.

I rode in the middle, sandwiched between the two of them, while she clung to a plastic bottle of locally made coconut oil.

We made our way up the hill, down the hill, past the beaches, the hotels, the health cafés, the massage parlors, the girl bars, the Muay Thai boxing gyms, until we arrived at our bungalow.

"How much did you pay for her?" I asked.

"Sixty bucks," he said. As with most prices, I was baffled by how cheap she was. Sixty bucks and she had no idea who we were, where we'd taken her, how long we'd keep her, what we'd do.

"How old are you?" I asked, flashing a dumb smile so she'd see I was a nice person.

"Nineteen," she answered in a voice I could barely hear. She smiled back.

I thought about myself at that age. Practically a virgin. Reading T. S. Eliot for the first time on my study abroad trip to Florence. Skipping class for gelato afternoons, riding trains through Europe. Weed shops in Amsterdam. Ice caves in Zermatt. The Louvre. The Coliseum. Would she ever know these kinds of places?

She seemed to know her way around our place. Into the bedroom and onto the bed.

I felt guilty when she removed her top. Guiltier when she obediently put her hands behind her back as I kissed and then suckled her small, brown, erect nipples. Even guiltier when she moved her fingers inside of me until I came.

River didn't say anything. He watched from the other side of the room. After I was satisfied, I got dressed and we drove her only halfway back, paying a taxi to finish our job because we were too ashamed to spend any more time with her. When we returned to the bungalow, I crawled back into bed and sobbed. There was the same old emptiness inside of me, and I was tired of looking at it.

"I think we should leave Thailand," he said, crawling in bed next to me. His heart thumped against my back.

"And go where?" I asked, feeling hopeless as I turned to face him. Looking into his eyes, I knew what I wanted. For us to work. Desperately. I wanted to put the past away, not just the things he'd done, but all the things I'd done and all the things I kept doing. I wanted to start fresh.

"I have an idea," he said.

◆

River and I decided to return to LA, but not for long. I introduced
him to my parents and showed him a few of the touristy sites—
the Hollywood sign, the Walk of Fame, In-N-Out Burger, Venice
Beach—but then we drove north to White Sulphur Springs, where
he'd enrolled me in something called the Hoffman Process. I was
wary about new age workshops and retreats after the disappointment of the tantra festival in Thailand, but River assured me this was
different. He had done the Process years ago in Australia and had
also signed himself up for a refresher course separate from mine.

The website for the Hoffman Process doesn't give much away,
and that's intentional. Participants are meant to embrace the mystery, walking in with an open heart and open mind, knowing only
that the weeklong retreat is designed to help them heal the past,
unlearn harmful habits, and build the life they want.

River and I separated—he to a friend's place in San Francisco
and I to a forty-five-acre retreat site in the heart of California's
wine country. I turned off my cell phone as instructed in the welcome packet and committed myself to this mysterious week. Un-
fortunately, just like the phone and internet, wine was also strictly
forbidden.

I checked in and settled into my cottage, shared with an angry
eighteen-year-old girl who nodded hello at me but showed no interest in connecting. That was fine. I left her there and walked over
to the dining area for dinner, where the other participants were
eating and making light conversation. There were about twenty of
us, all eyeing one another with uncertainty. It appeared that none
of us knew what we'd signed up for. Characteristically, I sat next
to the most attractive-looking guy there. He was wearing thick-
rimmed glasses and skinny jeans.

"What are you in for?" he asked, smiling.

I didn't know what to say because I wasn't really sure what to expect yet. I shrugged. "Curiosity, I guess? How about you?"

"I need to stop cheating on my wife," he answered, matter-of-factly.

I nodded. This was going to be intense.

◆

For one week, I did everything my four Process teachers suggested with one goal in mind: become somebody new. The Process entails a series of steps: becoming aware of our unhealthy patterns, tracing our patterns back to where we learned them (mainly through our parents or caregivers), learning how to cultivate compassion, and last, envisioning a bright new future.

Combining techniques that range from deep meditation and visualization to gestalt and group therapy, the Process is meant to condense a lifetime of psychoanalysis into a mere week. In his book *The 10 Secrets of 100% Healthy People*, Patrick Holford calls the Process "a psychological detox." Participants are busy from around 8:00 a.m. to 10:00 p.m. every day. Some of the work is highly physical, designed to help you purge repressed emotions so you emerge sweaty and exhausted, but clearer in the head. Crying and getting angry is not just welcome but encouraged, and you find yourself becoming more comfortable watching others work out their shit right in front of you so they no longer seem like strangers but other versions of your own messy self. And some of the work is deeply analytical, writing and thinking extensively about your past and how this past continues to shape your present.

One of the most terrifying, yet important techniques for me was the mere act of confession. I announced my deepest fears and secrets to the other participants. I didn't just announce them. I shouted them. I examined where I'd learned these fears and secrets, how I'd clung to them as my identity—that I was ugly, uninteresting, boring, unlovable, only good for sex, and probably not even *that good*—all along inventing a personality that didn't feel like the real me. The real me was kinder, calmer, curious. She was an adventurer, a writer, an artist. She possessed a gentleness and wanted desperately to connect with others. The real me was an optimist, a warrior, someone who believed in herself and her own innate goodness. She was lighthearted, passionate, and full of words and stories that she couldn't wait to share.

I traveled far back, through guided visualizations, to see myself at twelve years old, the most fragile time in my life. It was clear that *this* was the beginning. This was the origin of my hurt and I'd always known it. That's why I avoided the photo albums from these years or left the room if someone brought up a story about this time. But no matter how hard I tried to escape her, I still felt like that girl, never aged, never healed. It suddenly occurred to me that I didn't need to build somebody new; I needed to reach back and retrieve that little girl. I saw myself in the bathtub, lonely and afraid, using the sensation between my legs to escape the big, scary feelings I didn't know how to process. I felt the metal of my back brace cold and oppressive against my skin. I saw the terror in my eyes as I peered into a reflection that I was just beginning to despise.

I saw my baby sister coddled by my parents, and I resented her for taking them from me. I needed them. I also needed my brother, sucked into his teenage social life and less concerned with his awkward, back-braced little bother of a sister. I needed my friends at school, kids who obviously didn't know how to deal with what I must have looked like to them—some sad and disabled creature who didn't know how to use her own voice to ask for what she needed: to be loved.

I wrote down these memories on sheets of paper so I couldn't ignore them. I spoke them to my teachers and the other participants. And I kept speaking, even when I felt embarrassed or when I broke down in tears because I felt so sorry for myself. Yet nobody rolled their eyes and said what I feared most, "Get over it already. Move on. Your pain isn't important."

Instead, they all encouraged me to listen to that girl inside. Even though other people couldn't be there for her, *I* could be there for her. I was an adult now and I was strong enough to take care of her. I could be my own best friend, my biggest ally, my greatest romance.

And I could forgive everyone who'd ever let me down because they were hurting too. Everyone was hurting. I traveled back to see my parents as children and saw clearly where they'd learned their own patterns, which had helped me shape my own. I felt compassion for them in a way I'd never felt.

As we spoke our truths—all the injuries we'd survived and the lives we wanted to look forward to—the group grew closer and more affectionate with each other. We swam together, cried together, danced together, held each other close, and laughed until our bellies ached with joy. Even the angry eighteen-year-old girl who'd been closed off that first day became one of my closest confidantes in the group.

At one point in the week, I remember sitting out in one of the gardens watching several ants carrying a leaf across the ground beneath me. My head was free of distraction. I had the kind of clarity I'd wished for in meditation, only my eyes were open and I was fully awake and interested in my surroundings. I couldn't take my eyes off these ants. Small and vulnerable, but devoted to their work together. They were fascinating and they were enough. I didn't want anything else. I must have sat there for twenty minutes, content with the time passing. There was no drug in my system. No other place I wanted to be. No anxiety or boredom rising up in me. I felt peace and it was so familiar that I knew, without a doubt, this was my birthright. I was worthy.

ten

GIRL MEETS WOMAN

Here is what I have learned about trauma. Trauma can be ordinary. And when you have a chronic fear of ordinariness, you can convince yourself that your trauma actually isn't trauma at all. You'll listen instead to that loud voice inside your head saying, "Oh, you big crybaby. Stop making a big deal out of nothing. Some people have real problems." And so you'll blame a hundred other things—bad boyfriends, your parents, your city, yourself—except this terrible thing that happened to you. Why are we so resistant to place blame where it belongs? I think it's because we're scared of what comes next. Change. Healing. Living our lives. Becoming separated from all that we know.

Because that's exactly what happens. We do become separated from all we know. But instead of winding up alone, we find ourselves surrounded by truer friends. Instead of our environment being bleak and dreary as it has always been, there is light now. There is hope. In short, the things we fear are far superior to what we've grown accustomed to. Our new life actually feels like living, not riding shotgun to an erratic driver.

Habits loosen. Choices are possible again. We can be happy if we demand it.

If I were following a step-by-step guide on how to write an addiction memoir, this is where I'd tell you that I actively use all the tools I learned in the Hoffman Process, I attend SLAA meetings every week, and I haven't watched porn in years. I would tell you that I'm cured.

I wouldn't tell you about the time I got drunk on a work trip to New York and wound up at a peep show in Times Square. I wouldn't tell you about the time I masturbated next to the sleeping body of River just to give myself the rush of potentially getting caught. I wouldn't tell you about the strippers in Cabo. Or the strippers in LA.

But I'm not going to wait until I'm some pure and perfect person to consider my journey valuable enough to share with you. That person may never exist, and I'm OK with that. The person that does exist is flawed and insecure sometimes. She has cravings she doesn't give in to nearly as much as she used to, but she still has them. She might always have them. But what she doesn't have anymore—and this is huge, this is worth mentioning—is the desire to stay stuck. When shame creeps into her house like an alley cat, she pours some warm milk into a saucer so the poor thing can have a drink and then she makes herself a cup of tea so she can have a drink too.

When her woman voice is nowhere to be found and she runs to the mirror only to see a scared twelve-year-old girl staring back at her, she says hello and asks about her day.

She has learned the value of compassion and how to give that to herself when nobody else will.

Despite what all the self-help books say, I don't believe you need to love and accept yourself first before anybody can love and accept you. But I do believe you'll miss out on that love and acceptance if you aren't willing to follow suit and learn how to do it for yourself at some point. You might not know in this moment how you'll ever look into the mirror and see someone worthy of love, but you can start with a dream for it, a tiny dot of desire, which might just turn into action.

At the risk of sounding like a woman who was saved by a man, it's clear to me that meeting River, the man who eventually became my husband, changed the course of my life. But he's not some sort of guru. And his "saving" was only part of the saving I did and do for myself on what has become a day-to-day commitment to self-acceptance.

I won't say SLAA or therapy or self-help books or the Hoffman Process saved me either. Like River, these things offered opportunities to know myself better. And I slowly learned that it was safe to be vulnerable. Instead of being abandoned by judgment, indifference, or laughter, I received one standing ovation after the next. And I received even more acceptance than I knew existed in the world. From those around me. And from myself.

Once I was cracked open like that, appreciated for being raw, there was no way to close back up. I confessed every way I knew how, exposing myself at every given opportunity. I started writing essays about that little girl in the bathtub, how she first learned how to escape through the sensations that drowned out her suffering. I wrote about the hours wasted on the porn, on the men who didn't deserve me, on the men I didn't think I deserved. I wrote about the lies I told myself about myself—the painful chatter of the brain that will not quiet unless you let it seep out the way it wants to seep out.

In the past, I'd turned to writing as an attempt to make sense of what was happening in my life, to relieve my head from the racing thoughts by banishing them to the page. It had been a private activity except for that brief time in grad school where I toyed with the idea that maybe I could make the private public once I found a worthy subject. But what had I done or experienced that people would care about?

My first essay on sex addiction appeared on Salon.com in early 2014. I remember the fear and excitement that came over me when I received the email from then personal essays editor Sarah Hepola. She worked with me through several drafts, identifying the places where my reluctance was still obvious.

"There's an evasiveness here, like you don't want me to see you or don't want to be pinned down," she wrote. Then she helped me break through, dig deeper, and find the truth until the essay was the most honest thing I'd ever written. But did I really want strangers to know this much about me? What if my mom read it? What would everyone think?

River was full of encouragement. "This is what you need to be writing," he said. "It's real and it's brave."

After that first essay was published, my in-box flooded with letters. When the journalists called on me, asking me to share my story on radio shows and TV segments and in glossy magazine tell-alls, I accepted and spoke my truth, hoping that someone, somewhere, would feel less alone because of it. That maybe they'd be inclined to speak their truths too.

And when my readers wrote to me, reaching out for some connection, thanking me for speaking what they could not, I wrote back every time. These comrades ranged from a married father of four to a fourteen-year-old girl—both of them hooked on porn. They were more similar than what the research on sex and porn addiction would have you believe. And I didn't care how sick and twisted someone else might have thought them to be. I held them in the basket of my compassion and blanketed them in my humble but ever powerful *me too*—the best thing I have to offer.

◆

In October 2014, I found myself in a fancy-looking recording studio in midtown Manhattan, sitting across the table from the British playwright and author Tim Fountain. I was contacted by BBC Radio 4 to speak about the role of technology in addiction and ponder how the future might look as technology grew more sophisticated.

I showed up early, a nervous wreck. Though I'd been writing maniacally about the subject, using writing as a means of healing and connection, this radio interview was far more intimidating. The BBC was a big deal to me, and I'd somehow managed to trick them into thinking that I was some sort of authority on the topic.

But I didn't feel like an authority. Even though I was much kinder to myself, more open about my proclivities and keeping away from porn for the most part, I still didn't see myself as "cured" or "sober," and I feared I never would be. I knew recovery would be hard work, but I wasn't prepared for *how* hard it would be.

The BBC had paired us up because we were the same on one level: Tim and I had both admitted to having an unquenchable hunger for sexual pleasure. But we were also wildly different in another, more important regard: I saw myself as an addict intent on changing her ways, and Tim saw himself as a pleasure-seeker intent on staying the same.

"You've two ways of looking at it," he said. "I'm addicted to sex, or I'm just greedy and I like a lot of it. I like to say I'm just greedy and I like a lot of it." He smiled when he said this, completely confident with himself.

When I told him how sexual fantasy had ruled too much of my life, thinking that he might feel sorry for me and understand why I was intent on fixing myself, he kept smiling.

"Sexual fantasy is a vital part of somebody's sex life. The idea of 'making love' makes me shudder with boredom."

So I started feeling sorry for him. But also envious. Was he trying to change my mind? Did he doubt I had a problem? Did he doubt *he* had a problem? Where was his shame? His guilt? I didn't know much about his sexual history, but judging by the things he said and the hot younger man waiting for him outside the studio, I figured his sexual habits were far more suspect than mine.

Because he's a playwright, he told me that he saw my relationship to sex as a three-act drama. The first act is all that led me up to the present, the fiendish behavior and lack of control. The second act was having a relationship and putting away all my naughty, dirty habits. Then he said something that I've never forgotten.

"I just wonder if the happier medium—your third act— wouldn't be the combination of the two."

◆

Less than a year later, River and I were back in Thailand. We'd gotten married back in LA in a simple civil ceremony and were now living cheaply to pay off my student debt and save money for a house.

We met Nana at one of the girl bars where the young women stand around drinking Singha beer, flirting with the men who walk past. We chose that bar not because we wanted to pick up one of these girls but because nobody was using their pool table. I'd been getting better with a cue stick lately, and each win gave me a dose of self-confidence and bragging rights with which to torture my new husband.

Nana wore an off-the-shoulder, ruffled black blouse and jean shorts. Her huge back tattoo was in full view, a traditional *sak yant* tiger that symbolized power and fearlessness. *Sak yant* tattoos are all over the place in Thailand, but most common with Muay Thai fighters, prostitutes, and now tourists. The reason they are so common with Muay Thai fighters and prostitutes is because the *sak yant* is meant to bring protection to the bearer. Considering how dangerous those professions are, it makes sense.

Throughout the night, Nana and I couldn't stop looking at each other. She was hanging out with the other Thai girls, laughing and drinking, but unlike the other girls, she didn't call out to the men walking past. Every once in a while, one of the men would choose one of her friends and she'd switch seats or get another beer or walk past the pool table, smiling at us.

River and I smiled back at her and then at each other.

"Is she flirting with us?" I asked him.

"Not sure," he said. "Do you think she's a hooker?"

I shrugged.

After I'd beaten him twice, we asked our bartender for the bill. That's when Nana came over to us, introduced herself, and asked what we were up to next.

"Probably just going back to our hotel," I said. I was jittery. Unsure if she was a prostitute or not, I didn't know if she was going to offer us her services and I felt awkward declining when there was that part of me that wanted to say *yes, yes, yes*. I'd grown more accepting of that hungry voice inside my head, and this acceptance gave me power over my cravings, but it was still a challenge.

I'd already made up my mind about sleeping with prostitutes—it was depressing and I wanted no part in it. Unlike our last time in Thailand, I now felt equipped to make a choice in the matter simply by acknowledging my desire before it turned into an obsession. Seeing these women on the street didn't have to ruin me anymore—I could see them, want them, walk away from them, and get on with my day. This acknowledgment was the same technique I used on porn so I didn't wind up bingeing all day. I even used it when I felt compelled to lie, hide, blame, or act on any other compulsion that might lead to disaster or detachment.

"There's a dance party at another bar," she said. "You want to come?"

I looked at River, whose face told me I was in control. We would do whatever I wanted. Seeing us deliberating, Nana hurried us along.

"Here, I'll buy your drinks," she said, which seemed odd. What kind of prostitute pays for other people's drinks? Maybe she worked her clients differently.

A bit tipsy from the drinks, fascinated by her gesture, and high off my recent win at the pool table, I felt jovial enough to accept her invitation. "Why not?" I said. "Let's go dancing."

She led the two of us down the street, past the girl bars and late-night food vendors and darkened massage parlors, telling us a bit about her life. Her home was in Isaan in the northeast region of Thailand. River liked the music from there and he said so.

"And what do *you* like?" she asked, grabbing my hand.

You, you, you, I thought. But I just smiled in response.

At the bar, Nana and I bought each other tequila. River drank Coke. The three of us danced and laughed, our bodies loose and close. We kept dancing even when two drunk English guys got into a fight over a girl and started punching each other on the dance floor. We kept dancing even when the bartenders stopped serving drinks and they turned on the lights to shoo us out of the place. The only time we stopped dancing was when Nana's mouth landed on mine. And then I felt like we were floating.

Less than an hour later, we were back in our hotel room, the three of us taking a hot shower. While Nana and I soaped each other's bodies up, River stood behind me, kissing my neck and rubbing my shoulders. We didn't dry ourselves before moving to the bed, drenching the sheets and pillows while Nana and I explored each other's bodies and River caressed and watched, the three of us hungry but not desperate, indulgent but not greedy.

Afterward, we slept through the night, our bodies linked in a happy embrace. Before she kissed me on the mouth and left the next morning, I expected Nana to ask for payment, but she never did. She had spent the night with us because she desired us, and we had spent the night with her because we desired her. Maybe that's all it had to be.

◆

When I was a child, I was clumsy and fell down a lot. Whenever I got a bruise, I'd press the bruise lightly as its color faded, testing to see if I still felt any pain. I was fascinated by my body's ability to heal itself.

After the night with Nana, I tried to locate the bruise of my own shame, to press upon it and make sure it still lived there right beside this delicious moment I'd shared with her and River. I was so used to pain being synonymous with pleasure, but yet I couldn't force myself into feeling bad about this. No one had been coerced into anything they didn't want to do. Each of us had feasted, savored, and slept. There had been laughter, dancing, and kissing. There was no need to detach, cry, blame, or forget.

I thought to myself, *But I'm a sex addict. I should stay away from this sort of thing. This is dangerous.*

But it didn't feel dangerous at all. I wondered—had this been what Tim Fountain meant? Was I living my third act?

The Hoffman Process taught me to reclaim the girl I was at twelve, her insecurities, her self-hatred, her coping mechanisms, all of her. But what if I could go back to all the times in my life where I made a choice I'd later want to take back, and reclaim that girl too? What if I could go back and instead of taking back my "sins" and unlearning all the methods I'd learned to wreak havoc on my life, I took back the shame instead? What would my past look like then?

◆

One of my favorite photos from childhood is from a camping trip I took with my parents and older brother when I was nine years old. For three weeks, we drove up the California coast from LA to Yosemite, stopping in beach towns like Santa Barbara, Pismo Beach, Santa Cruz, and Monterey. We ate fresh oysters and drove across the Golden Gate Bridge in San Francisco. We visited the capitol building in Sacramento and soothed our muscles in Grover Hot Springs. And we stood inside the carved-out sequoias of Yosemite.

Of all the pictures of me inside towering trees, smiling up at waterfalls, or skipping through the waves, the one photo that resonates the most was taken inside the RV my parents rented, a big smile on my face, my hair permed, wearing a bright orange midriff T-shirt that reads, in big black letters: BOYS.

When my mom had taken me shopping for vacation clothes, I remember eyeing that shirt on the rack of other less provocative tops and needing it immediately. There was something important about it. Not only did it show off my young skin in such a liberating way, but it also announced to the world that I had an interest in

BOYS, big-lettered and bold, an indisputable personal statement. My mom took note of my enthusiasm and bought me the shirt, and I wore it all the time.

Many of the good feelings I get when I look at the photo probably have to do with that trip—spending all that time with my parents, who were free from work and atypically relaxed, roasting marshmallows and sitting around campfires, becoming acquainted with the vast beauty of California, but the other more poignant reason is what continues to fuel its appeal.

Wearing that shirt announced to the world in my own small way that I was a sexual being. As a child, I loved that I was making such a bold statement to the world, even if my mom and dad wouldn't imagine their little girl could be capable of sexual thoughts. I'd been noticing pleasant and mysterious sensations between my legs, and had enough knowledge to know that the sensations had to do with what happens between girls and BOYS.

I'm still drawn to that photo because it is one of my earliest memories of daring to be provocative, even when my parents probably just thought the shirt was "cute." Soon I'd turn ten and my sister would arrive. Then twelve, and I'd look into the mirror and cringe. Each year would bring with it a whole new set of reasons why I didn't deserve pleasure, why I should hate myself, why I should hide and pretend and escape. But in that photo, locked in time, as real and true as any other moment in my life, I knew what I wanted and I couldn't wait to say it. Look at me, BOYS. I'm a girl and I am sexual. I'm a girl and I have desires. I'm a girl and I am proud. Look at me looking at you.

ACKNOWLEDGMENTS

Willow Neilson, love of my life, greatest teacher, trusty copilot, best friend, and best human being that I know, thank you for loving me. The good times and even the not-so good times have enriched my life. Thank you for encouraging me to write this book, however delicate its subject matter. Thank you, especially, for parenting Frida with me. I honor both of you with my whole heart.

To my loving parents, Patricia and Gabriel Garza, thank you for never making me feel ashamed or embarrassed for wanting to tell this story and for never trying to talk me into getting "a real job."

A huge thanks to Heather Karpas, my brilliant and badass agent. I feel ridiculously lucky to know you. If it weren't for you, I don't think this book would have come to life for another twenty years. Or ever. Thank you for your enthusiasm, your honesty, and your willingness to push and push until I finished this thing. I am tremendously grateful.

To Gabe, Ashley, and Sunny, thank you for always being there, even when we are oceans apart.

To my editor, Cary Goldstein, thank you for believing in this work and in me.

Thank you also to Zachary Knoll for all of your helpful suggestions and to everyone at Simon & Schuster who played a role in bringing this book to life.

Thank you to Lis Harris, Patricia O'Toole, Stephen O'Connor, Amy Benson, Idra Novey, and the entire faculty at Columbia University's MFA Writing Program. You encouraged me to trust my voice and I am forever grateful for that.

To Amy Butcher and Nancy Rawlinson, thank you for working with me through several early drafts of what eventually became this book.

Thank you to Sarah Hepola for taking a chance on a mostly unpublished, budding essayist and helping me craft my first piece on sex addiction.

Thank you to Lisa Marie Basile for letting me write whatever I wanted at Luna Luna.

I owe a tremendous debt of gratitude to Uma Inder, Hope Matsuda, and Louise L. Hay for teaching me how to like myself.

Thank you to Jeanette and Volker Krohn for your encouragement and support.

Thank you to Hoffman Institute International for the important work you do.

To all the people I mention in this book—friends, lovers, classmates, teachers, acquaintances, heroes—thank you for the lessons you intentionally or unintentionally bestowed upon me.

And a very special thanks to Shannon Tweed, Pamela Anderson, Tommy Lee, Houston, Lupe Fuentes, and Luna Star. I'm not sure who I'd be without you.

ABOUT THE AUTHOR

Erica Garza's essays have appeared in *Salon*, *Narratively*, *BUST*, *Good Housekeeping*, and the *Los Angeles Review*, among other publications. She holds an MFA in nonfiction writing from Columbia University. Born in Los Angeles to a Mexican father and a Mexican-American mother, she has spent the majority of her adult life traveling and living abroad. She currently lives in Los Angeles with her husband and daughter.